The
Healing
Power of
Garlic,
Vinegar &
Olive Oil

Gayle Alleman, M.S., R.D.

Publications International, Ltd.

Gayle Povis Alleman, M.S., R.D., holds degrees in both alternative and conventional nutrition. She manages nutrition education programs and teaches nutrition in the community. She is also a freelance writer and speaker who focuses on food, nutrition, and health, and specializes in holistic nutrition.

Nutritional Analysis: Linda R. Yoakam, M.S., R.D., L.D.

The nutritional information that appears with each recipe was provided by the publisher. Every effort has been made to check the accuracy of these numbers. However, because numerous variables account for a wide range of values for certain foods, nutritive analyses in this book should be considered approximate. Slightly different results may be obtained by using different nutrient databases.

Louis Weber, CEO
Publications International, Ltd.
7373 North Cicero Avenue
Lincolnwood, Illinois 60712

Permission is never granted for commercial purposes.

ISBN-13: 978-1-4127-1321-4
ISBN-10: 1-4127-1321-8

Manufactured in U.S.A.

8 7 6 5 4 3 2 1

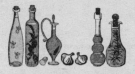

INTRODUCTION
FILL YOUR PANTRY WITH HEALING POWER

Garlic, vinegar, and olive oil—the mere mention of these three ingredients conjures images of fine, expertly crafted meals with complex layers of flavors and aromas. Garlic's pungency infuses everything it touches; the tart, and sometimes sweet, taste of vinegar lingers on your tongue; and the smooth, earthy taste of olive oil perfectly accents almost any ingredient in your kitchen.

But for all the ways they tantalize your taste buds, garlic, vinegar, and olive oil also do plenty of good work elsewhere in your body. Each helps the body battle some serious medical conditions. In their purest forms, these health boosters are products of nature, not of the laboratory. And, perhaps best of all, garlic, vinegar, and olive oil come in several varieties, which means you won't tire of finding ways to incorporate them into your diet.

Garlic has been used as a medicine for thousands of years, and it even had a role in the construction of the pyramids in Egypt. Modern science has shown that each clove of the teardrop-shape bulb is packed full of potent sulfur-containing compounds that help lower cholesterol levels, benefit the heart, fight infection, and possibly even help treat cancer.

People have used vinegar since ancient times as a remedy for everything from asthma, to headaches, to joint pain. Although vinegar seems to have suffered neglect at the hands of scientists in search of natural cures, some research points to its promise. Vinegar definitely helps the body absorb essential nutrients, including calcium. And some studies have shown that people living with type 2 diabetes, a condition that affects an estimated 20 million Americans, can use vinegar to help control blood sugar levels. Plus, vinegar can take the place of harmful ingredients in many recipes, lending flavor without adding fat or sodium.

Olive oil has been a staple for the Mediterranean people since ancient times. They savored its delightful taste and expert ability to blend the flavors of herbs and spices with foods. Now research is showing that consuming olive oil can help keep hearts and arteries in tip-top shape. This liquid gold is rich in monounsaturated fat, which helps lower cholesterol levels. Studies have shown that when people replace the unhealthy saturated fats in their diet with olive oil, they lose weight— even when consuming the same number of calories. And exciting research is under way to determine if olive oil can help prevent certain types of cancer.

You'll learn all this and more in *The Healing Power of Garlic, Vinegar & Olive Oil*. We've devoted two chapters to each of these three amazing ingredients. The first chapter in each pair explores the rich history of the ingredient and the modern-day efforts to uncover its healing power. You'll learn which nutrients the ingredient contains and get a few entertaining glimpses into the food's folklore and how people have used it throughout history.

The second chapter of each pair is packed with tips about how to identify and select the best varieties of the food to suit your needs, how to store it properly to maintain its healing properties, and how to prepare it so you're sure to make the most of its assets. Finally, at the back of the book, you'll find an imaginative array of recipes that will show you new ways to put these flavorful healers to use in your kitchen.

This book explores how these culinary favorites may help fight several serious health conditions, including heart disease, cancer, high blood pressure, and diabetes. Keep in mind, though, that the information in this book is intended to complement, not replace, proper medical care and the advice of a health-care professional. Be sure to speak with your physician regarding your individual medical concerns and treatments, including your use of garlic, vinegar, and olive oil. Then enjoy!

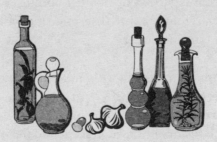

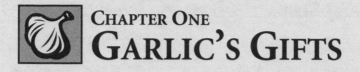

CHAPTER ONE
GARLIC'S GIFTS

The wonders of garlic have been with us for millennia. Writings from ancient Egypt, Greece, India, and China all make mention of the humble garlic clove. It has long been used in many cultures to improve health or transform meals into delicious, aromatic delights. Its ability to enhance flavor is undeniable, while the extent of its healing benefits continues to be revealed.

Garlic, or scientifically speaking, *Allium sativum*, is cultivated across the globe except in the polar regions. The bulb of this attractive plant contains more powerful sulfur compounds than does any other *Allium* species, such as onions and leeks. The garlic plant may have evolved to include these smelly sulfur compounds as a way of warding off foraging animals, invasive insects, and even soil-borne microorganisms such as bacteria and fungi. Yet these same compounds, which lend garlic its pungent aroma and delectable flavor as well as its medicinal qualities, are exactly the reason so many people are attracted to the bulb.

FABLES AND FOLKLORE

Garlic, which has been grown for more than 5,000 years, is one of the oldest cultivated plants in the world. Researchers think the ancient Egyptians were the first to farm garlic; in fact, the

The Stinking Rose
Didn't Bloom for Everyone

For all of garlic's uses, the history of the "stinking rose" is not all rosy. In certain times and places, people despised garlic. During his reign in the 14th century, King Alphonso of Castile ordered people to stay away from him if they had eaten garlic within the past month. Its alleged aphrodisiac qualities made garlic taboo for Tibetan monks. Ancient Indians believed garlic would lure people away from spiritual endeavors, so it was banned in certain sacred places. What's more, the upper classes among them felt it would be barbaric to eat such a "common people's food." The British considered garlic rank, and even Shakespeare mentioned it with disdain in several of his plays.

little bulbs helped power the building of the great pyramids. Hard-working slaves received a ration of garlic each day to improve their strength and ward off illness. And a mere 15 pounds of this ancient currency would buy a healthy male slave to add to the pyramid-building team. It seems fitting that garlic, a natural wonder with many healing and culinary properties, played a role in the creation of one of the wonders of the ancient world.

Ancient Egyptians bestowed many sacred qualities upon garlic. They believed it kept away evil spirits, so they buried garlic-shape lumps of clay with dead pharaohs. Archaeologists found preserved bulbs of garlic scattered around King Tut's tomb millennia after his burial.

The ancient Egyptians believed so strongly in the power of garlic to ward off evil spirits that they would chew it before making a journey at night. Garlic made them burp and gave them foul-smelling breath, creating a radius of odor so strong, they believed, that evil spirits would not penetrate it.

Ancient Greeks and Romans loved their garlic, too. Greek athletes and soldiers ate garlic before entering the arena or battlefield because they thought it had strength-enhancing properties. Roman soldiers ate garlic for inspiration and courage. Greek midwives hung garlic cloves in birthing rooms to repel evil spirits. Hippocrates, the ancient Greek known as the "father of medicine," prescribed garlic for a variety of ailments around 400 B.C. It was used to treat wounds, fight infection, cure leprosy, and ease digestive disorders. Other prominent Greeks used garlic to treat heart problems, as well.

Garlic's reputation as a medicinal wonder continued into the Middle Ages. It was used in attempts to prevent the plague and to treat leprosy and a long list of other ailments. Later, explorers and migrating peoples introduced this easy-to-grow and easy-to-carry plant to various regions around the world. The Spanish, Portuguese, and French introduced garlic to the Americas.

In many historic cultures, garlic was used medicinally but not in cooking. That might surprise us today, but were our ances-

GARLIC'S HISTORIC TARGETS

Garlic has been used throughout the ages to treat a long and varied list of ailments, including:

asthma
bladder infections
bronchitis
colds
colic
constipation
coughs
dandruff
diabetes
dysentery
earaches
eczema
fever
flatulence
flu
forgetfulness
gallbladder problems
graying of hair
hair loss
high blood pressure

indigestion
infections
infertility
insomnia
intestinal worms
liver problems
menstrual irregularities
paralysis
rabies
rheumatism
scabies
scorpion bites
seizures
sinus problems
tremors
tuberculosis
typhoid
ulcers
whooping cough

tors able to travel into the future to visit us, they would likely think us rather dense for our culture's general lack of appreciation for the bulb's healing qualities.

Traditionally, garlic bulbs were prepared in a variety of ways for medicinal purposes. The juice of the bulb might be extracted and taken internally for one purpose, while the bulb might be ground into a paste for external treatment of other health problems. In the minds of the superstitious, simply possessing garlic was enough to bring good luck and protect against evil—especially evil in the form of mysterious and frightening entities, such as sorcerers and vampires.

Legends convinced people that there were certain things over which vampires had no power, and garlic was one of them. However, it is only in European (and, by extension, American) folklore that vampires are powerless in the presence of garlic. The bulb apparently is not mentioned as a defensive tool against these infamous bloodsuckers in vampire legends from other parts of the world.

GARLIC MAKES THE HISTORY BOOKS

Garlic played its first starring role in modern medical treatment during World War I. The Russians used garlic on the front lines to treat battle wounds and fight infection, and medics used moss that was soaked in garlic as an antiseptic to pack wounds.

In the first part of the 20th century, garlic saw plenty of action off the battlefield, too. Even though penicillin was discovered in 1928, the demand for it among the general population often outstripped the supply, so many people reverted to treatments they had used with some success before, including garlic.

The pungent, ancient remedy has found its way to modern times. Herbalists have long touted garlic for a number of health problems, from preventing colds and treating intestinal problems to lowering blood cholesterol and reducing heart-disease risk. Garlic remedies abound—and scientific research has begun to support the usefulness of some of them.

Garlic's popularity today is due in part to the efforts of scientists around the world. They have identified a number of sulfur-containing compounds in garlic that have important medicinal properties.

If you were to look at or sniff an intact garlic clove sitting on a cutting board, you'd never suspect the potent aroma and healing properties within. Whack it with a knife, however, and you open a portal. Cutting, crushing, or chewing a garlic clove activates numerous sulfurous substances. When these substances come into contact with oxygen, they form compounds that have therapeutic properties. The most researched, and possibly the most medicinally powerful, of these potent compounds are allicin and ajoene.

A LITTLE HELP FOR YOUR HEART

The tiny garlic clove may play a big role in reducing the risk of heart disease, heart attacks, and stroke. How could such a simple herb have such powerful, far-reaching effects? To explore the answer and gain some appreciation for garlic's labors on our behalf, it's important to have a basic understanding of how the heart functions in sickness and in health.

Heart disease is the number one killer of Americans. The most common form of heart disease occurs when the arteries that deliver oxygen- and nutrient-rich blood to the heart become narrowed or clogged and lose their elasticity. Blood flow to the

A GUIDE TO HEART-DISEASE TERMS

Antioxidant: A substance that inhibits oxidation, a natural body process that causes cell damage. The body uses vitamins C and E as antioxidants. It also uses the minerals selenium and manganese to build potent antioxidant defense mechanisms, such as glutathione peroxidase and superoxide dismutase, to protect your cells.

Arteriosclerosis: A disease in which the arteries have thickened, hardened, and lost their elasticity, resulting in impaired blood flow. It develops in people who have high blood pressure, high cholesterol, diabetes, and other conditions or as the result of aging. It is also known as "hardening of the arteries."

Atherosclerosis: A type of arteriosclerosis characterized by plaque deposits on the interior walls of arteries.

Fibrinolysis: The body's natural process of breaking up blood clots.

Homocysteine: A sulfur-containing amino acid in the blood that has been linked to an increased risk of premature coronary artery disease, stroke, and blood clots in the veins.

Hypercholesterolemia: High levels of cholesterol in the blood.

Hyperlipidemia: High levels of lipids in the blood.

Lipids: Another word for fats. Includes all types of cholesterol and triglycerides.

Continued on page 14

Nitric oxide: In the human body, nitric oxide plays a role in oxygen transport, nerve transmission, and other functions. It also helps relax the lining of the blood vessels.

Oxidation: A chemical reaction between oxygen and another substance, sometimes resulting in damage to the substance. For instance, oxidized cholesterol damages the lining of arteries.

heart diminishes or may be cut off completely, starving the organ of oxygen. Without adequate oxygen, the heart can no longer work properly and heart cells begin to die.

Healthy arteries are similar to flexible tubes, wide open and able to contract and expand slightly as blood surges through with each heartbeat. When there is any injury to the inner lining of these vital tubes—such as damage caused by high blood cholesterol and triglyceride levels, high blood pressure, tobacco smoke, diabetes, and the aging process—the body tries to protect and heal the wounded area by producing a sticky substance to cover the damage.

This process is similar to the way we might use spackle to patch a small hole in drywall. But the sticky spackle the body produces to heal the wound causes fatty substances (including cholesterol), proteins, calcium, inflammatory cells, and other "debris" in the blood to stick to the vessel walls, forming plaque. As the plaque accumulates on the inner walls of the arteries, the arteries become less elastic, which leaves them vulnerable to even more injury. The gradual buildup of plaque also slowly narrows the inner diameter of the artery, and blood flow is hampered.

In addition, the plaque itself can crack, or bits of plaque can become dislodged. The body responds by sending platelets (particles in the blood that aid clotting) to form a clot around the plaque, further narrowing the artery. In some cases, the blood clot may completely block the flow of blood through the artery. Cells beyond the blockage that depend on a steady flow of oxygen from the blood can die. When this occurs in an artery that feeds the heart muscle (known as a coronary artery), it's called a heart attack. If this happens in a vessel that feeds the brain, the result is a stroke.

CARDIOVASCULAR DISEASE AND DIABETES

One of the well-known complications of diabetes, especially if the condition is not well controlled, is cardiovascular disease. Garlic may offer some protection to people with diabetes because of its antioxidant and anti-inflammatory properties.

CHOLESTEROL'S ROLE IN HEART DISEASE

Some cholesterol is necessary for normal body processes—it is a vital part of cell membranes, transports nutrients into and waste products out of cells, and is part of the structure of many hormones, among other functions—but too much of the wrong kind leads to trouble. A quick review of cholesterol will help you appreciate the beneficial role garlic might play in your heart's health.

HEART-HEALTHY GARLIC

Many studies have tried to determine whether—and how—garlic plays a role in keeping your ticker in tip-top shape. Research indicates that garlic plays a significant role in:

- Lowering blood pressure
- "Thinning" the blood
- Lowering triglycerides
- Lowering "bad" LDL cholesterol
- Breaking up blood clots
- Relaxing blood vessel walls and protecting them from damage

Scientists continue to research garlic's therapeutic effectiveness. Ongoing studies are gathering more data by changing the types and amounts of garlic used, the length of time participants use garlic, and the severity of participants' conditions.

Dietary cholesterol is a fatty substance, or lipid. When you eat cholesterol in food, as in meat, eggs, and cheese, your body breaks it down to digest it, then turns some of it back into cholesterol. Your body also makes cholesterol out of the solid fats (saturated fat and *trans* fat) in your diet.

Heredity also plays a role in the amount of cholesterol your body produces. Genetics determine whether your body makes a little or a lot of cholesterol from the fats you eat. If you have a

Know Your Numbers

Here are the optimal blood lipid levels from the National Heart, Lung, and Blood Institute (as of 2005):

- *Total cholesterol:* 200 milligrams of cholesterol per deciliter of blood (mg/dL) or less
- *LDL cholesterol:* 100 mg/dL or less
- *HDL cholesterol:* 40 mg/dL or more
- *Triglycerides:* 150 mg/dL or less

Note: Cholesterol levels are just one of several risk factors, including family history and smoking, that add up to determine your risk of heart disease. If you have one or more risk factors, you may need to aim for lipid levels lower than the standard ones listed here. Check with your health-care provider.

family history of high blood cholesterol, your body may make large amounts of the substance regardless of your eating and activity habits.

All this cholesterol is transported throughout your body via your internal highway—the bloodstream. There are several types of blood cholesterol. The most significant are:

LDL cholesterol. LDL stands for low-density lipoprotein. LDL is nicknamed "bad" cholesterol because as it flows through your arteries it has a tendency to stick to the artery walls and form plaque. As the plaque builds up, it narrows the arteries. Arteries lined with plaque are no longer flexible and elastic.

Instead, they are inflexible and "hard," which makes it more difficult for the heart to pump blood throughout the body, increasing your blood pressure. The more clogged the artery, the harder it is for blood to flow and deliver oxygen and nutrients to every part of the body.

HDL cholesterol. HDL stands for high-density lipoprotein. HDL carries the nickname "good" cholesterol because it works to eliminate excess blood cholesterol so it doesn't collect in the arteries and increase your risk for heart attacks and strokes. HDL carries cholesterol to the liver, where it is metabolized and then eliminated from the body. The higher your HDL level, the lower your chance of getting heart disease.

Triglycerides. Triglycerides are another form of lipid. Although they are not cholesterol, they do adversely affect your heart's health if you have too many in your blood. They can contribute to the thickening of artery walls. Your body manufactures triglycerides, and they are also present in food.

GARLIC'S IMPACT ON BLOOD CHOLESTEROL LEVELS

You've probably seen advertisements for garlic supplements and debated whether you should eat more garlic to improve your heart's health. Perhaps you've wondered if it's worth the odor or if it's only good for keeping vampires at bay. Does garlic really promote heart health, and if so, how?

Research on animals and humans in the 1980s and early 1990s seemed to indicate that garlic had much promise for lowering cholesterol. It appeared that garlic was able to lower total blood cholesterol in those who had high blood cholesterol (levels of 200 mg/dL or more). However, many of the studies included small numbers of patients and were short term, lasting just three months or less.

A number of more recent studies have tempered the initial enthusiasm about garlic's cholesterol-lowering effects. The National Center for Complementary and Alternative Medicine, a division of the National Institutes of Health (NIH), requested a thorough review of human studies that investigated garlic's ability to control cholesterol levels. The NIH released a paper in 2000 that concluded garlic did not alter HDL, but that it could significantly lower LDL cholesterol and triglycerides in the short term. Researchers determined that garlic had the greatest cholesterol-lowering effect in the first one to three months of garlic therapy. After six months, no further lipid reductions occurred.

Elevated cholesterol levels, however, contribute to heart disease over a long period of time. So based on this newer research, it would appear that although garlic may be a helpful addition to a cholesterol-lowering diet, it can't be relied on as the sole solution to high blood cholesterol levels.

Still, it's obvious that more research is needed. Indeed, the NIH statement in 2000 encouraged longer-term studies, as well as consideration of the type of garlic used. For example, there is some evidence that garlic must be cut or crushed to activate its health-promoting components. But the products tested in the various studies were not consistent. Some used raw garlic, while others used dried garlic or garlic oil; sometimes the raw garlic was cut, sometimes it was minced, and sometimes it was used whole. When dried garlic was used, it often was made into a powder and formed into tablets. It's also unknown whether

DIFFERENT FORMS OF GARLIC YIELD DIFFERENT RESULTS

One of the difficulties in comparing studies of garlic's effectiveness in humans is that there are many different forms of garlic used in the studies. One may contain more of an active ingredient than another. For example:

◆ *Fresh cloves of garlic—chopped or chewed:* These may impart the highest amount of allicin, but they have not been well studied yet.

◆ *Fresh cloves of garlic—swallowed whole:* These showed no therapeutic value in a limited number of studies that have been done.

◆ *Dehydrated garlic powder—made into tablets or capsules:* This form often provided some therapeutic value, but allicin content of these products varies within and among brands.

◆ *Enteric-coated garlic tablets:* These are treated so they do not dissolve until they reach your intestines, rather than your stomach. Some studies show that enteric-coated tablets don't dissolve soon enough to release the allicin they contain. This type of tablet usually prevents garlic odor on the breath.

◆ *Nonenteric-coated garlic tablets:* Tablets effective in studies were standardized to contain 1.3 percent allicin (more about the content of garlic supplements later). These may be more effective than the enteric-coated tablets, but they do cause garlic breath.

- **Aged garlic extract:** One of the active compounds in this form is ajoene. There have been conflicting results in studies of health benefits.
- **Garlic oil:** Shows little therapeutic value in studies.

garlic just stops being effective after several months or whether other factors in these studies influenced the findings.

THE BOTTOM LINE: GARLIC AND CHOLESTEROL

Although garlic may not be the blood-cholesterol miracle cure it was once promoted to be, and there are still plenty of questions that require answers, garlic does appear to have a healing role to play. A 2005 Mayo Clinic report gives garlic a grade of "B" for small reductions in blood cholesterol and LDL cholesterol over short periods of time (4 to 12 weeks). A "B" grade means there is good scientific evidence to support its use for that purpose. The Mayo Clinic reported the following findings from multiple studies:

- Supplements of nonenteric-coated tablets containing dehydrated garlic powder (standardized to 1.3 percent alliin) may reduce total cholesterol by up to 20 mg/dL for 4 to 12 weeks. The effects are unclear beyond 20 weeks.
- LDL may decrease by up to 10 mg/dL.
- Triglycerides may decrease by up to 20 mg/dL.
- HDL cholesterol levels are not significantly affected.

Mayo's report concluded that well-designed studies of longer duration and including more people might provide stronger evidence of garlic's cholesterol-reducing benefits. In the meantime, however, garlic is not likely to take the place of medications prescribed by a physician to lower blood cholesterol levels.

On the other hand, doctors often recommend that patients try lifestyle changes to lower cholesterol levels before or even along with drug therapy. Drugs often come with their own side effects—some merely unpleasant, others downright dangerous—and postponing or minimizing drug therapy with lifestyle changes can cut the risks of such side effects. Garlic's main drawback seems to be the odor it gives your breath and perspiration. Although garlic should never take the place of prescribed medications, including it more often in a cholesterol-lowering diet is easy, inexpensive, and enhances the flavor of your meals—especially those that are low in fat and sodium.

MORE WAYS THAT GARLIC WINS YOUR HEART

Luckily for us, nature packaged the equivalent of a chemical factory inside every little garlic clove. In addition to potent sulfur compounds such as allicin, garlic has other secrets in its heart-disease-fighting arsenal.

GARLIC'S ATTACK ON PLAQUE

Garlic contains several powerful antioxidants—compounds that prevent oxidation, a harmful process in the body. One of them is selenium, a mineral that is a component of glutathione peroxidase, a powerful antioxidant that the body makes to defend itself. Glutathione peroxidase works with vitamin E to form a superantioxidant defense system.

Other antioxidants in garlic include vitamin C, which helps reduce the damage that LDL cholesterol can cause, and quercetin, a phytochemical. (Phytochemicals are chemical substances found in plants that may have health benefits for people.) Garlic also has trace amounts of the mineral manganese, which is an important component of an antioxidant enzyme called superoxide dismutase.

Oxidation is related to oxygen, a vital element to every aspect of our lives, so why is oxidation so harmful? Think about when rust accumulates on your car or garden tools and eventually destroys the metal. That rust is an example of oxidation. Similarly, when your body breaks down glucose for energy, free radicals are produced. These free radicals start oxidizing—and damaging—cellular tissue. It's as if your bloodstream and blood vessels are "rusting out."

Antioxidants destroy free radicals, including those that are products of environmental factors, such as ultraviolet rays, air pollutants, cigarette smoke, rancid oils, and pesticides. The body keeps a steady supply of antioxidants ready to neutralize free radicals. Unfortunately, sometimes the number of free radicals can overwhelm the body's antioxidant stock, especially if we're not getting enough of the antioxidant nutrients.

When free radicals harm the cells that line your arteries, your body tries to mend the damage by producing a sticky spackle-like substance. However, as mentioned earlier, this substance attracts cholesterol and debris that build up within the arteries, causing progressive plaque formation. The more plaque in your arteries, the more your health is in danger.

CALCIUM: FRIEND OR FOE?

Your body needs calcium for building and maintaining strong bones and teeth, helping your muscles work properly, reducing your risk of colon cancer, and many other functions. So calcium is definitely a friend. What you don't want calcium to do is get involved with plaque formation. But don't think that cutting back on calcium will lower the risk of this harmful process.

Your body determines how it uses calcium, and you can't do much about it. If you avoid calcium-rich foods, your body will make up for the deficit by drawing calcium out of its "savings account"—your bones. This can leave you with weakened bones that are more susceptible to breakage and eventually osteoporosis, a disease in which bones become very thin and break easily.

Consume about 1,000 milligrams of calcium each day (an eight-ounce glass of fat-free milk has 300 milligrams of calcium) to preserve your bone bank of calcium. Prevent calcium-fueled plaque buildup in your blood vessels not by avoiding calcium but by eating less saturated and *trans* fat and eating more antioxidant-rich foods, such as fruits, vegetables, and garlic.

In addition, the cholesterol circulating through your arteries can be oxidized by free radicals. When LDL is oxidized, it damages the lining of the arteries, which significantly contributes to the buildup of plaque and the narrowing and hardening of the arteries.

Arteries, then, benefit greatly from the protection antioxidants provide. And garlic's ability to stop the oxidation of cholesterol may be one of the many ways it protects heart health.

Garlic also appears to help prevent calcium from binding with other substances that lodge themselves in plaque. In a UCLA Medical Center study, 19 people were given either a placebo or an aged garlic extract that contained S-allylcysteine, one of garlic's sulfur-rich compounds, for one year. The placebo group had a significantly greater increase in their calcium score (22.2 percent) than the group that received the aged garlic extract (calcium score of 7.5 percent). The results of this small pilot study suggest that aged garlic extract may inhibit the rate of coronary artery calcification. If further larger-scale studies confirm these results, garlic may prove to be a useful preventative tool for patients at high risk of future cardiovascular problems.

EASING THE PRESSURE

Research suggests that garlic can help make small improvements in blood pressure by increasing the blood flow to the capillaries, which are the tiniest blood vessels. The chemicals in garlic achieve this by causing the capillary walls to open wider and reducing the ability of blood platelets to stick together and cause blockages. Reductions are small—10 mmHg (millimeters of mercury, the unit of measurement for blood pressure) or less. This means if your blood pressure is 130 over 90 mmHg, garlic *might* help lower it to 120 over 80 mmHg. That's a slight improvement, but, along with some simple lifestyle adjustments, such as getting more exercise, garlic might help move your blood pressure out of the danger zone.

Preliminary studies indicate that garlic may also increase the production of nitric oxide. This chemical compound is produced in the lining of blood vessels, and it helps the vessels relax and allow blood to flow more freely. Research published in August 2005 in the *Proceedings of the National Academy of Sciences* indicates that some of the sulfur-rich compounds in garlic help the blood vessels relax and enlarge, lowering blood pressure and improving blood flow throughout the body.

THE BOTTOM LINE:
GARLIC AND HEART HEALTH

Garlic seems to deserve a spot on the battlefield in the fight against heart disease. Even if its lipid-lowering abilities are less extensive than once thought, it appears that garlic's antioxidant ability helps protect arteries from plaque formation and eventual blockage. Because garlic also appears to increase the nitric oxide in vessels and lower your blood pressure, it becomes even more valuable.

INFECTION FIGHTER

Garlic's potential to combat heart disease has received a lot of attention, but it should receive even more acclaim for its antimicrobial properties. Fresh, raw garlic has proven itself since ancient times as an effective killer of bacteria and viruses. Once again, we can thank allicin.

Laboratory studies confirm that raw garlic has antibacterial and antiviral properties. Not only does it knock out many common cold and flu viruses but its effectiveness also spans a broad range of both gram-positive and gram-negative bacteria (two major classifications of bacteria), fungus, intestinal parasites, and yeast. Cooking garlic, however, destroys the allicin, so you'll need to use raw garlic to prevent or fight infections.

ANTIMICROBIAL ACTIVITY

Garlic's infection-fighting capability was confirmed in a study conducted by researchers at the University of Ottawa that was published in the April 2005 issue of *Phytotherapy Research*. Researchers tested 19 natural health products that contain garlic and five fresh garlic extracts for active compounds and antimicrobial activity. They tested the effectiveness of these substances against three types of common bacteria: *E. faecalis*, which causes urinary tract infections; *N. gonorrhoeae*, which causes the sexually transmitted disease gonorrhea; and *S. aureus*, which is responsible for many types of infections that are common in hospitals. The products most successful at eradicating these bacteria were the ones with the highest allicin content.

Now garlic is being investigated to see whether it can help us battle microbes that are resistant to antibiotics. Can garlic go where current antibiotics cannot and knock out the resistant bacteria? Perhaps.

There are about as many versions of the four thieves' vinegar story as there are recipes for the concoction. One popular version, reported to be from the Parliament of Toulouse archives of 1628–1631, goes like this: Four thieves living in Marseilles, France, during the 17th century plagues were convicted of going to the houses of plague victims and robbing them, but the thieves themselves never became ill. How was this possible? In order to get a lesser sentence they revealed their secret—they protected themselves by consuming daily doses of a mixture that contained vinegar, garlic, and a handful of other herbs. Those in charge were so grateful that they hanged the four thieves, rather than burning them at the stake. That's gratitude for you!

One simple but meaningful demonstration of garlic's antibacterial power can be found in a study conducted at the University of California, Irvine. Garlic juice was tested in the laboratory against a wide spectrum of potential pathogens, including several antibiotic-resistant strains of bacteria. It showed significant activity against the pathogens. Even more exciting was the fact that garlic juice still retained significant antimicrobial activity even in dilutions ranging up to 1:128 of the original juice.

Is it possible that garlic can work alongside prescription medications to reduce side effects or to help the drugs work better? Results from several studies say yes.

In a Rutgers University study that used bacteria in lab dishes, garlic and two common antibiotics were pitted against certain antibiotic-resistant strains of *S. aureus* (a gram-positive bacteria) and *E. coli* (a gram-negative bacteria). Garlic was able to significantly increase the effectiveness of the two antibiotic medications in killing the bacteria.

Research done in Mexico City at a facility supported by the National Institutes of Health of Mexico also showed some interesting results. It extended previous research in rats that used aged garlic extract and various sulfur-containing compounds from garlic along with gentamicin, a powerful antibiotic that can cause kidney damage. When any of the garlic compounds was ingested along with gentamicin, kidney damage was diminished.

Next, researchers set about to determine whether garlic weakened the effectiveness of gentamicin. As it turns out, the exact opposite happened: Garlic actually *enhanced* the effect of gentamicin. These findings indicate that with the use of garlic, perhaps less gentamicin would be needed, and kidney damage could be minimized.

Judging by research conducted in lab dishes and animals, it appears that garlic is a strong defender against microbes, even against those that have developed a resistance to common antibiotics. It also appears that garlic enhances the effects of some traditional antibiotics. But does it stand up to the test in humans?

GARLIC'S
ANTI-INFLAMMATORY PROPERTIES

Inflammation is the body's reaction to an injury, irritation, or infection. The symptoms of inflammation include redness, swelling, and pain.

Whenever the body suffers an injury, it sends many substances to the site to begin the healing process and to fight off foreign invaders, such as bacteria that can cause infections. Inflammation is so vigorous in its duties that sometimes the surrounding tissues get damaged. This can occur at the site of a wound, inside blood vessels that have succumbed to an injury by oxidized LDL cholesterol, or in airways that are exposed to something that irritates them.

Certain complexes in garlic appear to help minimize the body's inflammatory response. By decreasing inflammation, garlic may lend a hand by doing the following:

◆ Protecting the inside of your arteries

◆ Reducing the severity of asthma

◆ Protecting against inflammation in the joints, such as in rheumatoid arthritis and osteoarthritis

◆ Reducing inflammation in nasal passages and airways, such as that associated with colds.

BATTLING THE BUGS WITHIN

Eating raw garlic may help combat the sickness-causing bugs that get loose inside our bodies. Garlic has been used internally as a folk remedy for years, but now the plant is being put to the test scientifically for such uses. So far, its grades are quite good as researchers pit it against a variety of bacteria.

For eons, herbalists loaded soups and other foods with garlic and placed garlic compresses on people's chests to provide relief from colds and chest congestion. Now the Mayo Clinic has stated, "preliminary reports suggest that garlic may reduce the severity of upper respiratory tract infection." The findings have not yet passed the scrutiny of numerous, large, well-designed human studies, so current results are classified as "unclear."

Can a garlic clove help stop your sniffles? A study published in the July/August 2001 issue of *Advances in Therapy* examined the stinking rose's ability to fight the common cold. The study involved 146 volunteers divided into two groups. One group took a garlic supplement for 12 weeks during the winter months, while the other group received a placebo. The group that received garlic had significantly fewer colds—and the colds that they did get went away faster—than the placebo group.

Garlic also may help rid the intestinal tract of Giardia lamblia, a parasite that commonly lives in stream water and causes giardiasis, an infection of the small intestine. Hikers and campers run the risk of this infection whenever they

FIGHTING THE COMMON COLD

Herbalists recommend chewing garlic and holding it in your mouth for a while before swallowing it to obtain the best dose of bacteria-fighting allicin. This may be rather difficult for children or for those who find garlic to be too spicy. As an alternative, mince a clove, let it sit for 10 to 15 minutes so the allicin can form, then stuff it into empty gelatin capsules (which you can purchase in the herb section of a natural foods store). Taking three cloves a day when you have a cold may help you feel better. If the raw garlic bothers your stomach, take the capsules with food that contains a little bit of canola oil or, better yet, olive oil.

Other folk remedies battle colds and chest congestion with a garlic poultice or plaster. To make one, put some chopped garlic in a clean cloth, thin washcloth, or paper towel. Fold it over to enclose the garlic. Pour very warm (but not hot) water over the wrapped garlic, let it sit for a few seconds, and then lightly wring it out. Place the wrapped garlic on the chest for several minutes. Reheat with very warm water and place on the back, over the lung area, for several minutes. Some herbalists also recommend placing the poultice on the soles of the feet.

Caution: Be careful not to let garlic come into direct contact with the skin. Cut garlic is so powerful that prolonged exposure to the skin may result in a burn.

drink untreated stream or lake water. Herbalists prescribe a solution of one or more crushed garlic cloves stirred into one-third of a cup of water taken three times a day to eradicate Giardia. If you're fighting giardiasis, be sure to consult your health-care provider, because it's a nasty infection, and ask if you can try garlic as part of your treatment.

Finally, in the January 2005 issue of *Antimicrobial Agents and Chemotherapy*, researchers reported the results of an investigation into whether fresh garlic extract would inhibit *C. albicans*, a cause of yeast infections. The extract was very effective in the first hour of exposure to *C. albicans*, but the effectiveness decreased during the 48-hour period it was measured. However, traditional antifungal medications also have the same declining effectiveness as time passes.

TREATING YEAST INFECTIONS

One of the traditional ways women have self-treated vaginal yeast infections is by carefully peeling a clove of garlic without nicking it, wrapping it in a small piece of gauze, and inserting it into the vagina overnight. The garlic is removed in the morning, and the treatment is repeated for the next several nights, until 24 hours after symptoms diminish. There hasn't been any scientific research done to confirm that this home remedy works, but many women have used it for yeast infection relief through the years.

EXTERNAL TREATMENTS

Garlic has many uses on the outside of the body, too. Applying a topical solution of raw garlic and water may stop wounds from getting infected. (Simply crush one clove of garlic and mix it with one-third of a cup of clean water. Use the solution within three hours because it will lose its potency over time.) A garlic solution used as a footbath several times a day is traditionally believed to improve athlete's foot.

A study conducted at Bastyr University, a natural health sciences school and research center near Seattle, showed that a garlic oil extract cured all warts it was applied to within two

GARLIC AND YOUR GUMS

Garlic may even help your gums stay healthy. In a study published in the July 2005 issue of *Archives of Oral Biology*, researchers concluded that garlic extract inhibits disease-causing bacteria in the mouth and may be valuable in fighting periodontitis, a serious gum disease. (Untreated gingivitis often leads to periodontitis, a condition in which the ligaments and bones supporting the teeth become infected and inflamed, ultimately resulting in tooth loss.)

This is exciting news because oral health can impact the rest of your body. For instance, disease-causing bacteria in your mouth can get into the bloodstream via bleeding gums, travel to your heart valve, and damage it.

TREATING BUG BITES

Some herbalists recommend treating insect bites with garlic. Here are some ways to do it (be careful with the first two options to avoid burning the skin):

- Rub a cut clove of garlic directly on the site.
- Mash a clove of garlic into a paste and apply.
- Make a quick "extract" of garlic. Crush some garlic, mix it with warm water, then use clean cotton swabs to apply the liquid to the insect bite.

weeks. A water extract of garlic was much less effective. In the same study, the garlic oil extract also proved useful in dissolving corns.

Using garlic oil extract appears to work better than the old folk remedy of tying or taping a slice of garlic to a wart. If the slice of garlic is bigger than the wart or moves just a bit, it blisters the healthy surrounding skin (of course, you have the same risk when using wart-removing products that contain acid). Garlic's phytochemical compounds are strong enough to create chemical burns, so always apply externally with caution and do not use on young children. One way you can protect the surrounding healthy skin is to smear petroleum jelly on it before you apply the garlic.

CANCER CRUSADER

Some scientists think garlic may be able to help prevent one of the most dreaded maladies—cancer. The Mayo Clinic has reported that some studies using cancer cells in the laboratory, as well as some studies with animals and people, have suggested that eating garlic, especially unprocessed garlic, might reduce the risk of stomach and colon cancers.

The National Institutes of Health's National Cancer Institute drew similar conclusions after reviewing 37 studies involving

CANCER-FIGHTING CLOVES

Crushing, chopping, or chewing garlic releases a host of cancer-fighting compounds, including some with names you might recognize and some that may not be familiar. They include:

- allicin
- alliin
- alline
- ajoene, a disulfide
- diallyl disulfide (DADS)
- diallyl sulfide (DAS)
- diallyl trisulfide (DAT)
- quercetin (a phytochemical that is a potent antioxidant)
- S-allylcysteine (SAC)
- selenium (a mineral that is part of an antioxidant complex made by the body)
- vitamin C (has proven antioxidant activity)

garlic and sulfur-containing compounds. Twenty-eight of those studies indicated garlic possessed at least some anti-cancer activity, especially toward prostate and stomach cancer. Because the studies in question were merely observational (they compared people who reported eating a lot of garlic to those who did not), more studies are needed.

Still, the research the National Cancer Institute reviewed found that it may not take much garlic to reap these anticancer benefits. Eating as few as two servings of garlic a week might be enough to help protect against colon cancer. Controlled clinical trials will help determine the true extent of garlic's cancer-fighting powers.

What gives garlic this wonderful gift? Several factors, including antioxidants and those same sulfur-containing agents we've discussed before, including allicin. (Antioxidants help protect cells from damage; continual cell damage can eventually lead to cancer.) Allicin appears to protect colon cells from the toxic effects of cancer-causing agents. For instance, when meat is cooked with garlic, the herb reduces the production of cancer-causing compounds that would otherwise form when meat is grilled at high temperatures.

Garlic's potential ability to decrease *H. pylori* bacteria in the stomach may help prevent gastritis (inflammation of the stomach lining) from eventually evolving into cancer. (*H. pylori* is most famous for its link to stomach ulcers, but it can also cause chronic gastritis.) Numerous studies around the world indicate that garlic's sulfur-containing compounds have the potential to help prevent stomach cancer.

The American Institute for Cancer Research (AICR), an organization that supports research into the roles diet and nutrition play in the prevention and treatment of cancer, has cited two large studies—one in China and the other in Italy— in which garlic intake was associated with lower death rates from stomach cancer. In addition, a Korean study indicated garlic consumption led to a lower risk of developing stomach cancer. And the AICR has reported that the Iowa Women's Health Study revealed that women had a lower risk of colon cancer if they ate garlic regularly. (The report did not define what amount and frequency constituted regular use.)

The amount of garlic you eat, along with the number of years you eat it regularly, may determine its ability to decrease cancer risk. This makes sense because cancer takes a long time to develop. In general, researchers suspect that garlic delivers anticancer benefits if you eat substantial amounts of it for three to five years or longer (again, the report did not define how much garlic should be eaten). That's when they begin to see a possible link in the reduction of laryngeal, gastric, colon, and endometrial (uterine) cancers.

Most studies do not show a reduction in breast cancer risk related to garlic intake. The data about whether garlic helps prevent development of prostate cancer is less definitive. And in a preliminary study that looked at consumption of fruits and vegetables, garlic appeared to be the only variable that might slightly decrease the risk of ovarian cancer; clearly, however, more studies are needed.

Garlic might defend against skin cancer when applied topically to tumors. In a study that appeared in the July 2003 issue of

GARLIC FOR WEIGHT CONTROL?

Studies performed on rats indicate that when fed allicin while on a sugar-rich diet, the rodents' blood pressure, insulin levels, and triglyceride levels all decrease. A study that appeared in the December 2003 issue of the *American Journal of Hypertension* showed other surprising results. The weight of the rats that were fed allicin either remained stable or decreased slightly. The weight of the rats in the control group increased. The researchers stated that, "allicin may be of practical value for weight control." Certainly, additional research needs to be done into this possible action of allicin, but it again demonstrates how wide-ranging garlic's benefits could be.

Archives of Dermatological Research, ajoene significantly shrunk skin cancer tumors in 17 out of 21 patients. The AICR has reported that in laboratory studies, the garlic compounds diallyl disulfide and ajoene protect against skin cancer.

Don't try treating skin cancer or unidentified/suspect skin lesions with garlic yourself, however. Skin cancer is a serious disease, and if you have it or suspect it, you should be following your physician's treatment guidelines. If you have a suspicious lesion, bring it to your physician's attention before using any home remedies.

A LOOK INSIDE A CLOVE

A clove of garlic a day is often the amount recommended for medicinal purposes. Garlic contains an array of nutrients, but vitamins and minerals aren't the only health-bestowing substances present. Phytochemicals, naturally occurring chemicals that plants produce, abound in garlic. Many of them contain sulfur and have been highlighted earlier. Here is a look at some of the essential nutrients within a single clove.

CALORIES	4.5
MACRONUTRIENTS	
Carbohydrate	<1 g
Fat	<1 g
Protein	<1 g
Fiber	0.06 g
VITAMINS	
Thiamin (B_1)	0.01 mg
Riboflavin (B_2)	0.01 mg
Niacin equivalents	0.05 mg
Vitamin B_6	0.04 mg
Vitamin C	0.94 mg
Folate	0.09 mcg
MINERALS	
Calcium	5.43 mg
Copper	0.01 mg
Iron	0.05 mg
Magnesium	0.75 mg
Manganese	0.05 mg
Phosphorus	4.59 mg
Potassium	12.03 mg
Selenium	0.43 mcg
Sodium	0.51 mg
Zinc	0.03 mg

g=grams mg=milligrams (0.001 grams) mcg=micrograms (0.000001 grams)

GARLIC'S SAFETY

Garlic is safe for most adults. Other than that special aroma garlic lends to your breath and perspiration, the herb has few side effects. However, you should know about a few cautions:

◆ If you are allergic to plants in the Liliaceae (lily) family, including onions, leeks, chives, and such flowers as hyacinth and tulip, avoid garlic. People who are allergic to garlic may have reactions whether it's taken by mouth, inhaled, or applied to the skin.

◆ People anticipating surgery or dental procedures, pregnant women, and those with bleeding disorders should avoid taking large amounts of garlic on a regular basis due to its ability to "thin" the blood, which could cause excessive bleeding. Taking blood thinners such as warfarin (brand name Coumadin) or aspirin and other nonsteroidal anti-inflammatory drugs (such as ibuprofen or naproxen) along with garlic is not recommended unless you first discuss it with your health-care provider so dosing adjustments can be made. To be safe, if you have any questions about your use of garlic, talk with your health-care provider.

◆ Garlic interferes with medications other than anticoagulants. Garlic may interact with and affect the action of birth control pills, cyclosporine (often prescribed for rheumatoid arthritis), and some other medications. It also interferes with certain HIV/AIDS antiviral medications, reducing their effectiveness. Talk with your health-care provider and/or pharmacist if you take prescription medications and regularly eat large amounts of garlic or take any type of garlic supplement.

EAR INFECTION THERAPY

Garlic extract added to olive oil is an age-old remedy for ear infections. Herbalists recommend slightly heating the oil, adding a very small amount of sliced garlic, letting it sit for a few minutes, and then straining it thoroughly before putting a couple of drops into the infected ear. There must be absolutely no garlic particles in the oil.

Before you place the oil in the ear, place a few drops on the inside of your arm and let it sit for several minutes to be sure that it is not strong enough to burn your arm (either because of the temperature of the oil or the amount of garlic essence present). If it passes the test, put a few small drops into the infected ear. Make a fresh batch for each treatment.

It's safest to check with your health-care provider before trying this home remedy, and it is essential if you have or have ever had a ruptured eardrum.

◆ Nursing women may find that garlic gives their milk an "off" flavor that the baby may reject, resulting in shorter nursing times.

◆ Consuming large amounts of garlic can irritate the stomach lining and possibly cause heartburn, abdominal pain, flatulence, diarrhea, or constipation. Go easy with garlic if you have a sensitive stomach.

- If applied directly to the skin, garlic can cause burns. Be especially careful using raw garlic on children's skin.

If the strong odor garlic gives your breath, perspiration, and skin bothers you, consume less of it.

THE SKINNY ON SUPPLEMENTS

Fresh, naturally grown raw garlic is best, but if you can't get enough of it into your diet, here is the scoop on supplements.

As noted in several of the research studies mentioned, not all garlic supplements consistently have the amount of allicin claimed on the label when they undergo testing. There are many possible variables, including differences in the garlic itself, growing conditions, amounts and types of fertilizer, type of garlic, the processing methods used, and quality control during manufacturing.

This remains a problem with assessing research on garlic—do the commercial garlic preparations contain what they say they do? Which compounds do they really have and how much is there in the supplement you're taking?

Supplements are typically made by slicing garlic and drying it at low temperatures to prevent the destruction of alliinase, the enzyme that turns alliin into the disease-fighter allicin. It is then pulverized into a powder and formed into tablets. In order to meet the standards set by the U.S. Pharmacopeia (the group that develops the quality standards for prescription and over-the-counter drugs and dietary supplements sold in the United States), the powder must contain at least 0.3 percent alliin.

Because manufacturers process and label their supplements differently, shopping for garlic supplements can be confusing. Some tablets do not contain any allicin, but rather alliin, which is converted to allicin. Other tablets contain both alliin and allicin. And some supplement labels may have an "allicin potential" or "allicin yield" statement. This refers to the amount of allicin that *could* be formed when alliin is converted, not how much allicin is *actually* formed.

In addition, because the enzyme alliinase is destroyed by the strong acidic conditions in the stomach, most supplements are "enteric coated" to keep them from dissolving until they reach the small intestine. Most tablets tested, though, produce only a little allicin under these tough conditions, and the tablets often take too long to dissolve. The better measurement is "allicin release." This discloses how much allicin the supplement actually produces under conditions similar to those found in the digestive tract. However, only a few manufacturers list this measurement on their labels.

With all this in mind, you should start by looking for the "standardization" statement on a label when choosing a garlic supplement—but even this isn't a foolproof guarantee. When a product is "standardized" it is supposed to have a certain amount of a specific ingredient. For instance, a product that says, "standardized to contain 1.3 percent alliin" means that every pill in every bottle should contain at least 1.3 percent alliin. Unfortunately, this is not always the case, but a product that carries the USP (U.S. Pharmacopeia) seal follows set methods to help ensure standardization.

Allicin is not the only active compound in garlic, but the other compounds are typically not standardized. Thus, you often don't know everything you're getting when purchasing a supplement.

Which kind of supplement is best? Dried garlic powder is considered to have effects similar to those of fresh, crushed garlic. Other types of supplements, such as oils from crushed garlic, aged garlic extract in alcohol, and steam-distilled oils seem to contain less allicin and perhaps less of other active compounds than the dried powder.

When shopping for a garlic supplement, look for one that indicates it is standardized to contain at least 1.3 percent allicin. In the United States, pharmacy-grade garlic contains 0.3 percent (powdered form) to 0.5 percent (fresh, dried form) allicin. Avoid enteric-coated or time-release tablets because these may not dissolve soon enough in your digestive tract to make use of the allicin.

How Much Should You Take?

Large scientific boards make several recommendations about garlic dosage. The Mayo Clinic cites the European Scientific Cooperative on Phytotherapy's recommendation for prevention of atherosclerosis as 3 milligrams to 5 milligrams allicin (3,000 micrograms to 5,000 micrograms allicin) or one clove or 0.5 gram to 1 gram of dried powder.

THE BOTTOM LINE

- Aim for about 5 milligrams of allicin per day.

- Use supplements that state the amount of "allicin release" rather than "allicin yield" or "allicin potential."

- When reading supplement labels, note that the amount of allicin is often listed in micrograms (mcg) rather than milligrams (mg). There are 1,000 micrograms in 1 milligram, so a supplement that contains 5,000 micrograms of allicin has 5 milligrams of allicin, which meets the European Scientific Cooperative on Phytotherapy's recommendation of 3 milligrams to 5 milligrams of allicin.

- A supplement may contain 500 milligrams of dried garlic bulb, which is equal to 0.5 gram. This falls into the low end of the World Health Organization's recommendation for dried garlic powder. Remember that dried powder contains just a small amount of allicin. Other compounds make up the rest of the tablet.

The World Health Organization recommends 2 grams to 5 grams of fresh garlic, 0.4 gram to 1.2 grams of dried garlic powder, 2 milligrams to 5 milligrams of garlic oil, 300 milligrams to 1,000 milligrams of garlic extract, or some other formulation that yields the equivalent of 2 milligrams to 5 milligrams (2,000 to 5,000 micrograms) of allicin daily.

GO TO THE CLOVE

Rather than fussing over garlic supplements that may or may not contain what they claim, just enjoy the heady aroma and flavor of fresh garlic in the foods you eat. You'll always know you're getting the best—and the most potent—allicin you can when you add garlic to foods. Consider this:

◆ A typical garlic clove weighs about 3 grams.

◆ The amount of alliin in an average clove ranges from 24 milligrams to 56 milligrams.

◆ A standard clove will produce about 2.5 milligrams to 4.5 milligrams of allicin per gram of fresh weight when crushed. This means you'll get 7.5 milligrams to 13.5 milligrams of allicin from one typical clove that weighs 3 grams.

What else on your plate delivers such a punch of healing power in such a small and flavorful package?

CHAPTER TWO
GARLIC: A CULINARY DELIGHT

The type of garlic you choose and how you prepare and use it combine to determine its healing properties and flavor. This chapter will show you how to make the most of your garlic, and enjoy every bit—and bite—of it.

Beautiful garlic braids decorate many kitchens. Some are adorned with peppers or dried flowers while others sport a country ribbon. But garlic's role in the kitchen shouldn't be limited to wall decor. With a peel and a chop, garlic adds an aroma and flavor that few ingredients can match. This modest herb enlivens a kitchen, enchanting at least three of our senses.

Chefs all over the world put garlic to work in their kitchens. And a little clove really gets down to business. Not only does garlic boost the flavor of other foods but it also possesses many healthful and healing properties.

Garlic plays the role of star or supporting cast member equally well, whether it's used in appetizers, main courses, side dishes, drinks, or even desserts. Don't be shy about adding it almost anywhere. If you're not sure how, where, and when to use garlic, keep reading! The tips in this section and the recipes later in the book will help you get to know garlic in the most intimate and delicious ways.

GARLIC VARIETIES

Garlic, garlic, hanging on the wall, which of you is the best of all? The first step to a perfect meal is selecting the ideal bulb from the more than 400 species and varieties of garlic. *Allium sativum* is the most common type of garlic; it is the one you'll typically find in the grocery store and is often called "culinary" garlic. Fortunately, this is the species that also offers the most healing properties.

You might occasionally find *Allium ursinum* in specialty or farmer's markets. *Allium ursinum* is a type of wild garlic native to Northern Europe that does not possess the same healing properties as *Allium sativum*. You might also come across *Allium vineale*, a garlic with very small cloves that is commonly called "crow garlic." This variety is nothing more than a weed.

Allium sativum has two subvarieties: softneck and hardneck. The two types have similar healing properties because they belong to the same species, but they differ in flavor, clove size, shelf life, and use.

SOFTNECK GARLIC

Softneck garlic is the type you'll most likely see in the produce section of your grocery store. Its name comes from the multi-layered parchment that covers the entire bulb, continues up the neck of the bulb, and forms a soft, pliable stalk suitable for braiding. Its papery skin, or sheath, is a beautiful creamy white color.

Softneck garlic typically has several layers of cloves surrounding the central portion of the garlic bulb. The outermost layer's cloves are the stoutest; the cloves of the internal layers become smaller closer to the center of the bulb. Of the several types of softneck garlic, two are most abundant:

Silverskin garlic. This easy-to-grow variety has a strong flavor and stores well when dried—it will last nearly a year under the right conditions. The Creole group of silverskin garlics has a rose-tinted parchment.

Artichoke garlic. Artichoke garlic has a milder flavor and may have fewer and larger cloves than silverskin. You can store it as long as eight months. Artichoke garlic may occasionally have purple spots or streaks on its skin, but don't confuse it with purple stripe garlic, a hardneck variety that has quite a bit of purple coloring.

HARDNECK GARLIC

Unlike softneck garlic, hardneck varieties do not have a flexible stalk. When you buy this type of garlic, it will typically have an extremely firm stalk protruding an inch or two from the top of the bulb.

Hardneck garlic sends up scapes from its central woody stalk when it is growing. A scape is a thin green extension of the stalk that forms a 360-degree curl with a small bulbil, or swelling, several inches from its end. Inside the bulbil are more than 100 tiny cloves that are genetically identical to the parent bulb beneath. Many people call these "flowers," but they are not really blooms. If left on the plant, the scape will eventually die and fall over, and the tiny cloves will spill onto the ground. However, most never make it that far.

Garlic Lovers Unite!

The annual Gilroy Garlic Festival in Gilroy, California, invites you to celebrate this "palate-pleasing herb" during the last full weekend of July. The festival debuted in 1979 and has grown into an incredible event. In 2005, the festival hosted nearly 130,000 people, involved the work of 4,000 volunteers, and raised more than $300,000 for 170 local charities.

This famous festival also boasts a garlic cook-off that begins in December with a call for great garlic recipes and ends with finalists preparing their dishes in front of the crowd in July. Entertainment, arts, crafts, and dozens of delectable garlic dishes await festival attendees. For more information, visit the festival Web site at www.gilroygarlicfestival.com.

Can't make it to California? Take heart—there are many smaller garlic festivals, too. An Internet search for "garlic festivals" will yield hundreds of events, some of which are probably in your area.

Cutting off the scapes keeps the plant's energy from forming the bulbil and therefore encourages larger bulbs. But don't throw out the scapes. They can be a delicious ingredient in your cooking.

There are three main types of hardneck garlic:

Rocambole. This variety has a rich, full-bodied taste. It peels

GARLIC'S FAMILY TREE

Family: Liliaceae

The lily family contains more than 4,000 species, including common garden flowers such as daylilies and trillium. Some botanists now classify *Alliums* into their own family, *Aliaceae*.

Genus: *Allium* (includes garlic, onions, leeks, scallions, chives, and shallots)

Species: *Allium sativum* (cultivated garlic)

Varieties: hardneck and softneck

Subvarieties:

HARDNECK	SOFTNECK
rocambole	artichoke
porcelain	Asiatic
purple stripe	turban
marbled purple stripe	silverskin
glazed purple stripe	silverskin Creole

easily and typically has just one set of cloves around the woody stalk. It keeps for up to six months.

Porcelain. Porcelain garlic is similar to rocambole in flavor and typically contains about four large cloves wrapped in a very smooth, white, papery sheath. People often mistake porcelain garlic for elephant garlic (discussed later) because its cloves are so large. Porcelain garlic stores well for about eight months.

Purple stripe. This hardneck variety is famous for making the best baked garlic. There are several types of purple stripe, all with distinctive bright purple streaks on their papery sheaths. Purple stripe garlic keeps for about six months.

Another member of the *Allium* clan, elephant garlic (*Allium ampeloprasum*), may look like a good buy because it is so large, but its flavor is very bland. Elephant garlic tastes more like a leek; in fact, its garlic flavor is slight and its healing properties are inferior to those of other garlic varieties. Use elephant garlic more like a vegetable than a flavorful herb.

THE BRIGHTEST BULB

Once you've decided which variety of garlic to use, consider the following tips to find that perfect bulb:

◆ Select bulbs that are completely dry.

◆ Choose bulbs whose cloves are plump and firm.

◆ Look for plenty of papery sheath.

◆ Avoid soft or crumbly cloves; spongy or shriveled cloves; bulbs or cloves with green shoots (they are past their prime); and preminced garlic, which has a weak flavor.

GROWING GARLIC

It's easy to grow your own garlic. It's hardy, tolerates cold weather well, and does not need pampering. Whether in a garden or a patio pot, garlic grows well under most conditions and requires little maintenance.

Many gardeners, especially those in northern climates, plant their garlic in October. Others prefer to do it on the shortest day of the year—the winter solstice in December. Planting in the fall lengthens the growing time so bulbs get a jump start on spring and can grow larger. Some gardeners in more southern climates prefer to plant garlic four to six weeks before the date of the last frost.

Garlic is robust enough to survive the frigid months, but if the winter seems too cold or the snow doesn't form a thick enough blanket over the plants, you can cover the bulbs and emerging shoots with straw or other mulching material for insulation.

You can try planting the garlic you buy from your local grocery store, but some grocery store garlic is treated with a sprout inhibitor that disrupts the natural growing cycle. If you don't know whether your store-bought garlic is treated this way, visit a plant nursery or garden center to purchase naturally grown garlic that is suitable for gardening. If you prefer to try your hand with specialty garlics, visit a garden center or check a seed catalog.

How to Plant

To plant garlic, gently remove the outer skin from the entire bulb and separate the individual cloves, taking care not to damage them. (Leave in place the thin papery skin that covers each clove.) Choose about eight to ten of the largest cloves from the outside of the bulb for planting.

Place the cloves in the ground, tip up, in a place that gets about six hours of direct sunlight per day. Garlic needs to grow quickly to form large bulbs, and full sun fosters fast growth. You'll also want to be sure the area in which you plant will not become waterlogged in winter.

Plant Pals

Many gardeners firmly believe in companion planting—the idea that some plants prefer certain kinds of "company" to others. When these plants grow next to one another, they seem to fare better and have improved flavor. Some plants emit odors that protect others against particular pests. Scientists aren't completely certain why these relationships work (most are not scientifically proven), but many long-time gardeners swear by them.

Garlic deters pests, so plant it liberally throughout the garden. It may discourage aphids, nibbling insects, and even snails and slugs. As an added bonus, planting garlic near herbs is said to enhance their essential oils.

Avoid planting garlic near peas, potatoes, or legumes, however, because these plants don't do well when planted next to garlic.

Work the soil about ten inches deep, adding organic matter and perhaps even sand to improve drainage. Bury the cloves in this loose, fertile soil so the tips are about two inches beneath the surface of the soil and the cloves are four to six inches apart. Apply a weak organic fertilizer every two weeks or so. Water the plants regularly so the soil is moist but not overly soggy, and pluck out weeds that would otherwise compete for nutrients and possibly overgrow the garlic.

Your Guide to Planting Garlic

When: Plant either in the fall or four to six weeks before the last frost.

Where: Plant in loose, fertile, well-drained soil that gets about six hours of direct sun daily.

How: Set cloves point up, two inches deep and at least four inches apart.

Water: Provide ample water throughout the growing season and less as plants mature.

Fertilizer: Apply mild organic fertilizer every two weeks.

Harvest: When tops turn yellow and dry out, dig up the entire plant.

Garlic prefers hotter and drier conditions as it matures. If you water the garlic less frequently near the end of the growing season, it will dry out a bit and its flavor will be better. Of course, the amount of water your garlic needs depends on your area's climate, so keep a close eye on your soil.

Harvesting Garlic

It's time to harvest your garlic when the green tops dry out and turn yellow-brown. This is typically about three to four months into the growing season—late summer or early fall. Some gardeners prefer to harvest their garlic on the longest day of the year—the summer solstice in June. Harvest too early, and you get small bulbs. Harvest too late, and the bulbs may split. This indicates that they have already started their next growing season and diminishes their culinary quality.

Before you harvest all your plants, carefully dig up one bulb and examine it. Check its size, and count the layers of papery skin. If the bulb seems well formed, the cloves are plump, and there are about three layers of papery covering, harvest your crop. If there are four or more layers, let the plants grow a bit longer. When you're ready to harvest, use a small garden trowel to loosen the soil around each bulb. Then dig up the entire plant and shake off loose soil.

Some gardeners save part of their crop for planting again. Others believe that doing so heightens the risk of disease and results in smaller bulbs the next year. Because you can easily buy garlic to plant at a garden center, there may not be a need to save any cloves, unless you cultivate unusual varieties.

Storage

Storing your garlic in favorable conditions helps to maintain its healing properties and flavor. Properly stored garlic can last for months, ensuring that you always have some on hand for the next recipe.

"Young wet," or "new season," garlic is an immature garlic that is harvested in early summer. Immature garlic needs to be stored in the refrigerator and used within a week or so. It has a fresh, mild flavor and can substitute for onions and leeks or lend a subtle garlic flavor to a recipe. Some cooks consider this the best, most flavorful garlic. As an added bonus, it may be more easily digested than dry garlic. Experiment with some of this "fresh" garlic and see how you like it.

WATCH FOR MOLD

You should occasionally check your stored garlic—all cloves should be firm when you gently press them. If a clove becomes soft or shows signs of mold, remove it from the bulb, being careful not to nick the other cloves. If a clove begins to sprout, remove the green sprout and use the clove right away because flavor deteriorates after sprouting.

You'll need to dry your home-grown garlic before you store it for a prolonged time. After harvesting, carefully wash the bulb and roots. Let the garlic dry in a shady, well-ventilated, moisture-free area for a week or more. You can hang the freshly harvested bulbs from their stalks if you like. Thoroughly drying garlic bulbs develops and concentrates their flavor, so don't rush the process. Once dry, trim or break off the roots and rub off the outer layer of parchment. If you've grown softneck garlic, consider braiding it for an attractive storage option.

Whole bulbs of store-bought garlic will keep for several months or more when stored at room temperature in a dry, dark place that has ample air circulation. Keep in mind, however, that garlic's lifetime decreases once you start removing cloves from the bulb. Storing garlic uncovered, such as in a wire-mesh basket inside your cupboard or beneath a small overturned clay pot, is ideal. You can also store garlic in a paper bag, egg carton, or mesh bag. Just be sure there is plenty of dry air and little light to inhibit sprouting. To avoid mold, do not refrigerate or store garlic in plastic bags.

If you've prepared more garlic than you need for a particular recipe, you can store minced garlic in the refrigerator in an airtight container. Although the most active sulfur compound diminishes within a few hours, refrigeration will slightly slow the process. Use refrigerated garlic as soon as possible. Some people are tempted to freeze garlic, but this is not recommended because its texture changes, as does its flavor.

GARLIC IN THE KITCHEN

The first thing to remember about cooking with garlic is the difference between bulbs and cloves. The average teardrop-shape garlic bulb is about two inches wide and two inches tall. It typically contains about 10 to 20 individual cloves about the size of your thumbnail. Most recipes call for one or more *cloves*, not *bulbs*.

EASY PEELING

To easily peel garlic, slice off each end of a clove. Then, turn your broad chef's knife sideways so the flat side is parallel to your cutting board and the sharp edge is facing away from you. Place your knife this way on top of the clove and give the blade a quick pop with the heel of your hand to lightly crush the garlic clove (you don't want to mash it). The papery skins then rub off easily.

If you're going to peel many garlic cloves at once, drop them into boiling water for 10 to 20 seconds. Then plunge them into cold water. The skins will slide right off between your thumb and forefinger.

To separate the individual cloves from the bulb, place the bulb on a flat surface. Use the heel of your hand to apply firm but gentle pressure at an angle. The parchment layers will separate, allowing you to carefully remove as many cloves as you need. Then, tenderly remove the thin covering on each individual clove. Most people reach for the plumpest cloves, but the smaller cloves have a more intense flavor.

THE FLAVOR OF FORCE

Whether you rule garlic with a gentle or firm hand determines the amount and type of flavor you get. Here are some taste tips:

- ◆ Gently peel and use cloves whole to impart just a hint of garlic flavor.
- ◆ Slice cloves lengthwise for mild flavor or for those long-cooking dishes.
- ◆ Mince cloves for medium flavor or for your quick-cooking dishes.

Firmly push cloves through a garlic press for the strongest flavor. If you don't have a garlic press, put your knife to work and finely chop the garlic. Remember, the smaller the pieces, the more pungent the flavor. Sprinkle the chopped garlic with a bit of salt, because salt pulls out liquid from the chopped garlic. Then firmly rub the salted chopped garlic with the side of your knife blade, further crushing it.

Because one of garlic's most beneficial ingredients, allicin, is partially destroyed by cooking, you'll get the greatest health boost if you use it raw or only lightly cooked when you can. However, cooking garlic forms other healthy sulfur compounds, so you still receive benefits when you cook it. Plan ahead so you can cut, crush, or chop your garlic and let it sit for 15 minutes or more before using it to activate the enzymes that turn alliin into allicin.

GIDDY FOR GARLIC AROUND THE GLOBE

Garlic adds the spice of life to foods in countries all around the world. Along with ginger and onions, garlic flavors many of the foods of Southeast Asia. Teamed with tahini, it makes Middle-Eastern foods dining delights. Combined with chili peppers, garlic adds spark to Latin cuisine. To bring garlic's robust flavor and health benefits to your own kitchen, try some of the recipes we've collected for you later in this book.

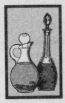

CHAPTER THREE
VERSATILE VINEGAR'S REWARDS

Vinegar has been valued for its healing properties for about as long as garlic has, and like garlic, vinegar has found its way from the apothecary's shelf to the cook's pot. Today, it can continue to play that dual role, taking the place of less health-ful dietary ingredients and helping to regulate blood sugar levels while entertaining our taste buds with its tart flavor.

There seems hardly an ailment that vinegar has not been touted to cure at some point in history. And while science has yet to prove the effectiveness of many of these folk cures, scores of people still praise and value vinegar as a healthful and healing food. So let's take a look at the history of vinegar, the healing claims made for it, and what science does and doesn't have to say about those claims. Along the way, we'll discover why vinegar deserves a place in every healthy kitchen.

VINEGAR'S HUMBLE BEGINNINGS

To understand the historical origins of vinegar, it helps to know a little something about how vinegar is "born." The following overview will help you understand the creation process, although you'll find a more detailed discussion of how the many varieties of vinegar are produced in chapter four.

Early Wines and Vinegars

Scientists believe wine originated during the Neolithic period (approximately 8500 B.C. to 4000 B.C., when humans first began farming and crafting stone tools) in Egypt and the Middle East. Large pottery jugs dating back to 6000 B.C. that were unearthed in archeological digs possessed a strange yellow residue. Chemical analysis revealed the residue contained calcium tartrate, which is formed from tartaric acid, a substance that occurs naturally in large amounts only in grapes. So the traces strongly suggested the jugs were used to make or hold wine.

Considering the slow grape-pressing methods used at that time and the heat of the desert environment, grape juice would likely have fermented into wine quite quickly. Likewise, the wine would have turned to vinegar rapidly, if conditions were right.

So how did these ancient people—who had only recently (in evolutionary terms) begun planting their own food and fashioning tools—manage to understand and control fermentation enough to prevent all their wine from turning to vinegar before they could drink it? Based on evidence found in archeological excavations, scientists believe that the first winemakers used jars with clay stoppers that helped control the fermentation process.

Continued on page 64

A complete analysis of the residue left in those ancient wine jugs also showed the presence of terebinth tree resin, which acts as a natural preservative and therefore would have helped slow the transformation of wine into vinegar. In Neolithic times, terebinth trees grew in the same area as grapes, and their berries and resin were harvested at the same time of year. So it's quite plausible that some of the berries or resins may have inadvertently become mixed with the grape harvest. Still unclear is whether the ancient winemakers ever made the connection between the resins and the delayed conversion of wine into vinegar and began purposely adding the tree berries to their wine.

Vinegar is a dilute solution of acetic acid that results from a two-step fermentation process. The first step is the fermentation of sugar into alcohol, usually by yeast. Any natural source of sugar can be used. For example, the sugar may be derived from the juice, or cider, of fruit (such as grapes, apples, raisins, or even coconuts); from a grain (such as barley or rice); from honey, molasses, or sugar cane; or even, in the case of certain distilled vinegars, from the cellulose in wood (such as beech).

What you have at the end of this first phase, then, is an alcohol-containing liquid, such as wine (from grapes), beer (from barley), hard cider (from apples), or another fermented liquid. (The alcoholic liquid used to create a vinegar is generally reflected in the vinegar's name—for example, red wine vinegar, white wine vinegar, malt vinegar, or cider vinegar.)

In the second phase of the vinegar-production process, certain naturally occurring bacteria known as acetobacters combine the alcohol-containing liquid with oxygen to form the acetic-acid solution we call vinegar. Acetic acid is what gives vinegar its sour taste. Although time-consuming, this second phase of the process will happen without human intervention if the alcoholic liquid is exposed to oxygen long enough.

Thus, it is not surprising that the first vinegar was the result of an ancient accident. Once upon a time, a keg of wine (presumably a poorly sealed one that allowed oxygen in) was stored too long, and when the would-be drinkers opened it, they found a sour liquid instead of wine. The name "vinegar" is derived from the French words for "sour wine."

Fortunately, our resourceful ancestors found ways to use the "bad" wine. They put it to work as a cure-all, a food preservative, and later, a flavor enhancer. It wasn't long before they figured out how to make vinegar on purpose, and producing it became one of the world's earliest commercial industries.

The use of vinegar as medicine probably started soon after it was discovered. Its healing virtues are extolled in records of the Babylonians, and the great Greek physician Hippocrates reportedly used it as an antibiotic. Ancient Greek doctors poured vinegar into wounds and over dressings as a disinfectant, and they gave concoctions of honey and vinegar to patients recovering from illness. In Asia, early samurai warriors believed vinegar to be a tonic that would increase their strength and vitality.

Vinegar continued to be used as a medicine in more recent times. During the Civil War and World War I, for example, military medics used vinegar to treat wounds. And folk traditions around the world still espoused vinegar for a wide variety of ailments. Natural-healing enthusiasts and vinegar fans continue to honor and use many of those folk remedies.

A CORNUCOPIA OF CLAIMS

The folk- and natural-healing claims made for vinegar through the ages have been almost as plentiful and varied as those made for garlic. Even in the current era of high-tech medicine, some proponents of natural healing still encourage traditional uses of vinegar. They have also added certain newly recognized or newly defined (within the past hundred years or so, that is) medical conditions to the list of health concerns for which they recommend vinegar.

Other present-day vinegar fans view it as an overall health-boosting, disease-fighting tonic and recommend mixing a teaspoon or tablespoon of cider vinegar with a glass of water and drinking it each morning or before meals. (Apple cider vinegar is the traditional vinegar of choice for home or folk remedies, although some recent claims have been made for the benefits of wine vinegars, especially red wine vinegar. Unless otherwise specified, though, the vinegar we'll be referring to in the rest of this chapter is apple cider vinegar.)

Perhaps most amazingly, vinegar is heralded as a potential healer of many of today's most common serious ailments. Devotees believe vinegar can help prevent or heal heart disease, diabetes, obesity, cancer, aging-related ailments, and a host of

VINEGAR TO THE RESCUE?

Apple cider vinegar has long been touted as a natural remedy for an amazing array of ailments, although there's little hard scientific evidence available to support many of its purported healing benefits. Vinegar has been used to treat the following conditions through the ages:

INTERNAL USES

appetite and digestive problems
asthma
constipation
cough and colds
depression
diarrhea
dizziness
fatigue
food poisoning
gallstones and kidney stones
headache
heartburn and hiccups
high blood pressure
high blood cholesterol
kidney and bladder problems
metabolism problems
osteoporosis
poor blood clotting
poor circulation
sore throat
upset stomach
urinary tract infections
yeast infections

EXTERNAL USES

age spots and liver spots
athlete's foot
dandruff
dry hair
ear infections and
    blockages
hay fever
hearing problems
insect stings and bites
insomnia
joint pain
leg cramps
nasal congestion
skin problems, such as
    eczema and rashes
strained muscles
sunburn
tired, sore eyes

other conditions. They say it is full of vitamins, minerals, fiber, enzymes, and pectin and often attribute vinegar's medicinal effects to the presence of these ingredients. Among the specific claims made for apple cider vinegar are that:

- **It reduces blood cholesterol levels and heart-disease risk.** Apple cider vinegar fans say it contains pectin, which attaches to cholesterol and carries it out of the body, thus decreasing the risk of heart disease. In addition, many vinegar proponents say it is high in potassium, and high-potassium foods play a role in reducing the risk of heart disease by helping to prevent or lower high blood pressure. Calcium is also an important nutrient for keeping blood pressure in check, and as you will learn shortly, vinegar is sometimes promoted as having a high calcium content. Many also claim vinegar helps the body absorb this essential mineral from other foods in the diet.

- **It treats diabetes.** Apple cider vinegar may help control blood sugar levels, which helps to ward off diabetes complications, such as nerve damage and blindness. It also might help prevent other serious health problems, such as heart disease, that often go hand-in-hand with diabetes.

- **It fights obesity and aids in weight loss.** Some marketers proclaim that apple cider vinegar is high in fiber and therefore aids in weight loss. (Fiber provides bulk but is indigestible by the body, so foods high in fiber provide a feeling of fullness for fewer calories.) A daily dose is also said to control or minimize the appetite. (Ironically, some folk traditions advise taking apple cider vinegar before a meal for the opposite effect—to stimulate the appetite in people who have lost interest in eating.)

- **It prevents cancer and aging.** Apple cider vinegar proponents declare it contains high levels of the antioxidant beta-carotene (a form of vitamin A) and therefore helps prevent cancer and the ill effects of aging. (Antioxidants help protect the body's cells against damage from unstable molecules called free radicals; free-radical damage has been linked to various conditions, including coronary heart disease, cancer, and the aging process.)

- **It prevents osteoporosis.** Advocates say apple cider vinegar releases calcium and other minerals from the foods you eat so your body is better able to absorb and use them to strengthen bones. Vinegar allegedly allows the body to absorb one-third more calcium from green vegetables than it would without the aid of vinegar. Some fans also say apple cider vinegar is itself a great source of calcium.

Based on these claims, apple cider vinegar certainly seems to be a wonder food. And it's understandably tempting to *want* to believe that some food or drug or substance will make diabetes, obesity, cancer, and osteoporosis go away with little or no discomfort, effort, or risk.

However, as a wise consumer, you know that when something sounds too good to be true, it almost certainly is. So when it comes to your health—especially when you're dealing with such major medical conditions—it's important to take a step back and look carefully at the evidence.

A Closer Look at the Claims

With such dramatic claims made for it, you would think that vinegar would be high on the lists of medical researchers

COMPLEMENTARY RESEARCH PRIORITIES

The NCCAM studies substances that hold possible promise in treating a health condition because they exhibit some type of active compound. An active compound can be a vitamin, mineral, or phytochemical—anything in a food, herb, or other natural substance that has some kind of therapeutic effect on the body.

The organization's list of research topics includes cardiovascular disease, disorders of the digestive tract, respiratory diseases (including colds and asthma), and obesity.

searching for the next breakthrough. Yet in the past 20 years, there has been very little research about using vinegar for therapeutic health purposes.

Granted, a lack of supporting scientific research is a common problem among many natural and alternative therapies. But even the National Center for Complementary and Alternative Medicine (NCCAM), a division of the U.S. government's National Institutes of Health that was created specifically to investigate natural or unconventional therapies that hold promise, has not published any studies about vinegar, despite the fact that there has been renewed interest in vinegar's healing benefits recently.

So without solid scientific studies, can we judge whether vinegar provides the kinds of dramatic benefits that its promoters and fans attribute to it? Not conclusively. But we can look at the claims and compare them to the little scientific knowledge we do have about vinegar.

Those who have faith in apple cider vinegar as a wide-ranging cure say its healing properties come from an abundance of nutrients that remain after apples are fermented to make apple cider vinegar. They contend that vinegar is rich in minerals and vitamins, including calcium, potassium, and beta-carotene; complex carbohydrates and fiber, including the soluble fiber pectin; amino acids (the building blocks of protein); beneficial enzymes; and acetic acid (which gives vinegar its taste).

These substances do play many important roles in health and healing, and some are even considered essential nutrients for human health. The problem is that standard nutritional analysis of vinegar, including apple cider vinegar, has not shown it to be a good source of most of these substances.

Take a look at the table on the next two pages—it shows the results of a nutritional analysis of an apple compared with the nutritional breakdown of two different amounts of apple cider vinegar. One tablespoon of apple cider vinegar per day is the typical therapeutic dose recommended, so the nutrients found in this amount of the vinegar are shown in the second column of the table. Just to be sure that the small amount of vinegar in a tablespoon isn't the sole explanation for the apparent lack of nutrients, the table also includes the nutritional analysis of a larger amount (half a cup) of vinegar. You'll notice that even at that higher amount, vinegar does not appear to include significant amounts of most of the nutrients that are claimed to be the source of its medicinal value.

To put all this information into some context, the column at the far right in the table shows the daily amounts needed by a typical adult who consumes 2,000 calories per day. (Requirements haven't been established for some of the other substances that are often cited as contributing to vinegar's beneficial effects.)

Nutrient	One medium apple, raw (2¾ inch diameter)	1 Tbsp. apple cider vinegar	½ cup apple cider vinegar	Daily amount needed by avg. adult
Calories	72	3	25	2,000
Carbohydrate	19.06 g	0.14 g	1.11 g	130 g
Fat	0.23 g	0 g	0 g	65 g (max.)
Protein	0.36 g	0 g	0 g	46 g (women) 56 g (men)
Fiber	3.3 g	0 g	0 g	25 g (women) 38 g (men)
Minerals				
Calcium	8 mg	1 mg	8 mg	1,000 mg
Iron	0.17 mg	0.03 mg	0.24 mg	18 mg (women) 8 g (men)

Nutrient	One medium apple, raw (2³/₄ inch diameter)	1 Tbsp. apple cider vinegar	¹/₂ cup apple cider vinegar	Daily amount needed by avg. adult
Magnesium	7 mg	1 mg	6 mg	320 mg (women) 420 mg (men)
Phosphorus	15 mg	1 mg	10 mg	700 mg
Potassium	148 mg	11 mg	87 mg	4,700 mg
Sodium	1 mg	1 mg	6 mg	1,500 mg
Zinc	0.06 mg	0.01 mg	0.05 mg	8 mg (women) 11 mg (men)
Copper	0.037 mg	0.001 mg	0.01 mg	0.9 mg
Manganese	0.048 mg	0.037 mg	0.298 mg	1.8 mg (women) 2.3 mg (men)
Selenium	0 mcg	0 mcg	0.1 mcg	55 mcg

Source: U.S. Department of Agriculture, Agricultural Research Service. 2005.
USDA National Nutrient Database for Standard Reference, Release 18.
Nutrient Data Laboratory Home Page, www.ars.usda.gov/ba/bhnrc/ndl.
Note: g = grams, mg = milligrams, mcg = micrograms.

As you can see, the one milligram of calcium in one tablespoon of apple cider vinegar does not come close to the
300 milligrams of calcium in eight ounces of milk, as some
promoters of apple cider vinegar claim. In fact, it supplies only

a tiny fraction of the 1,000 milligrams a typical adult needs in a day. Vinegar also contains little potassium.

In terms of pectin, the type of soluble fiber that is said to bind to cholesterol and help carry it out of the body, apple cider vinegar contains no measurable amounts of it or of any other type of fiber. So it would seem that pectin could not account for any cholesterol-binding activity that vinegar might be shown to have.

Do apple cider vinegar's secrets lie in the vitamins it contains? No. According to the USDA, apple cider vinegar contains no vitamin A, vitamin B6, vitamin C, vitamin E, vitamin K, thiamin, riboflavin, niacin, pantothenic acid, or folate.

What about some of the other health-boosting substances that are alleged to be in vinegar? According to detailed nutritional analyses, apple cider vinegar contains no significant amounts of amino acids. Nor does it contain ethyl alcohol, caffeine, theobromine, beta-carotene, alpha-carotene, beta-cryptoxanthin, lycopene, lutein, or zeaxanthin.

How Vinegar Can Help

So if vinegar doesn't actually contain all the substances that are supposed to account for its medicinal benefits, does that mean it has no healing powers? Hardly. As mentioned, so little research has been done on vinegar that we can't totally rule out many of the dramatic claims made for it. Although we know vinegar doesn't contain loads of nutrients traditionally associated with good health, it may well contain yet-to-be-identified phytochemicals (beneficial compounds in plants) that would

REMEDIES FOR MINOR AILMENTS

Vinegar's potential for treating or preventing major medical problems is of interest to almost everyone. But it also has been cherished as a home remedy for some common minor ailments for centuries. Although they're not life-or-death issues, these minor health problems can be uncomfortable, and there is often little modern medicine can offer in the way of a cure. So you may want to give vinegar a shot to determine for yourself if it can help. (It's always best when trying any remedy for the first time to run it past your doctor to be sure there is no reason you should not try it.)

Stomach upset. To settle minor stomach upset, try a simple cider vinegar tonic with a meal. Drinking a mixture of a spoonful of vinegar in a glass of water is said to improve digestion and ease minor stomach upset by stimulating digestive juices.

Common cold symptoms. Apple cider vinegar is also an age-old treatment for symptoms of the common cold. For a sore throat, mix one teaspoon of apple cider vinegar into a glass of water; gargle with a mouthful of the solution and then swallow it, repeating until you've finished all the solution in the glass. For a natural cough syrup, mix half a tablespoon apple cider vinegar with half a tablespoon honey and swallow. Finally, you can add a quarter-cup of apple cider vinegar to the recommended amount of water in your room vaporizer to help with congestion.

Continued on page 76

Itching or stinging from minor insect bites. In the folk-lore of New England, rural Indiana, and parts of the Southwest, a vinegar wash is sometimes used for treating bites and stings. (However, if the person bitten has a known allergy to insect venom or begins to exhibit signs of a serious allergic reaction, such as widespread hives, swelling of the face or mouth, difficulty breathing, or loss of consciousness, skip the home remedies and seek immediate medical attention.) Pour undiluted vinegar over the bite or sting, avoiding surrounding healthy skin as much as possible.

Athlete's foot. One way to eliminate athlete's foot (or other fungal infection) is to create an environment that is inhospitable to the fungus that causes the condition. The Amish traditionally use a footbath of vinegar and water to discourage the growth of athlete's foot fungus. To try this remedy, mix one cup of vinegar into two quarts of water in a basin or pan. Soak your feet in this solution every night for 15 to 30 minutes, using a fresh solution each night. Or, if you prefer, mix up a solution using one cup of vinegar and one cup of water. Apply the solution to the affected parts of your feet with a cotton ball. Let your feet dry completely before putting on socks and/or shoes.

account for some of the healing benefits that vinegar fans swear by. Scientists continue to discover such beneficial substances in all kinds of foods.

But beyond that possibility, there appear to be more tangible and realistic—albeit less sensational—ways that vinegar can help the body heal. Rather than being the dramatic blockbuster cure that we are endlessly (and fruitlessly) searching for, vinegar seems quite capable of playing myriad supporting roles—as part of an overall lifestyle approach—that can indeed help us fight serious health conditions, such as osteoporosis, diabetes, and heart disease.

INCREASING CALCIUM ABSORPTION

If there is one thing vinegar fans, marketers, alternative therapists, and scientists alike can agree on, it's that vinegar is high in acetic acid. And acetic acid, like other acids, can increase the body's absorption of important minerals from the foods we eat. Therefore, including apple cider vinegar in meals or possibly even drinking a mild tonic of vinegar and water (up to a tablespoon in a glass of water) just before or with meals might improve your body's ability to absorb the essential minerals locked in foods.

Vinegar may be especially useful to women, who generally have a hard time getting all the calcium their bodies need to keep bones strong and prevent the debilitating, bone-thinning disease osteoporosis. Although dietary calcium is most abundant in dairy products such as milk, many women (and men) suffer from a condition called lactose intolerance that makes it difficult or impossible for them to digest the sugar in milk. As a result, they may suffer uncomfortable gastrointestinal symptoms, such as cramping and diarrhea, when they consume dairy products. These women must often look elsewhere to fulfill their dietary calcium needs.

Dark, leafy greens are good sources of calcium, but some of these greens also contain compounds that inhibit calcium absorption. Fortunately for dairy-deprived women (and even those who do drink milk), a few splashes of vinegar or a tangy vinaigrette on their greens may very well allow them to absorb more valuable calcium. Don't you wish all medications were so tasty?

CONTROLLING BLOOD SUGAR LEVELS

Vinegar has recently won attention for its potential to help people with type 2 diabetes get a better handle on their disease. Improved control could help them delay or prevent such complications as blindness, impotence, and a loss of feeling in the extremities that may necessitate amputation. Also, because people with diabetes are at increased risk for other serious health problems, such as heart disease, improved control of their diabetes could potentially help to ward off these associated conditions, as well.

With type 2 diabetes, the body's cells become resistant to the action of the hormone insulin. The body normally releases insulin into the bloodstream in response to a meal. Insulin's job is to help the body's cells take in the glucose, or sugar, from the carbohydrates in food, so they can use it for energy. But when the body's cells become insulin resistant, the sugar from food begins to build up in the blood, even while the cells themselves are starving for it. (High levels of insulin tend to build up in the blood, too, because the body releases more and more insulin to try to transport the large amounts of sugar out of the bloodstream and into the cells.)

Over time, high levels of blood sugar can damage nerves throughout the body and otherwise cause irreversible harm. So one major goal of diabetes treatment is to normalize blood sugar levels and keep them in a healthier range as much as possible. And that's where vinegar appears to help.

It seems that vinegar may be able to inactivate some of the digestive enzymes that break the carbohydrates from food into sugar, thus slowing the absorption of sugar from a meal into the bloodstream. Slowing sugar absorption gives the insulin-resistant body more time to pull sugar out of the blood and thus helps prevent the blood sugar level from rising so high. Blunting the sudden jump in blood sugar that would usually occur after a meal also lessens the amount of insulin the body needs to release at one time to remove the sugar from the blood.

A study cited in 2004 in the American Diabetes Association's publication *Diabetes Care* indicates that vinegar holds real promise for helping people with diabetes. In the study, 21 people with either type 2 diabetes or insulin resistance (a prediabetes condition) and eight control subjects were each given a solution containing five teaspoons of vinegar, five teaspoons of water, and one teaspoon of saccharin two minutes before ingesting a high-carbohydrate meal. The blood sugar and insulin levels of the participants were measured before the meal and 30 minutes and 60 minutes after the meal.

Vinegar increased overall insulin sensitivity 34 percent in the study participants who were insulin-resistant and 19 percent in those with type 2 diabetes. That means their bodies actually became more receptive to insulin, allowing the hormone to do its job of getting sugar out of the blood and into the cells. Both blood sugar and blood insulin levels were lower than normal in the insulin-resistant participants, which is more good news. Surprisingly, the control group (who had neither diabetes nor a prediabetic condition but were given the vinegar solution) also experienced a reduction in insulin levels in the blood. These findings are significant because, in addition to the nerve damage caused by perpetually elevated blood sugar levels, several chronic conditions, including heart disease, have been linked to excess insulin in the blood over prolonged periods of time.

More studies certainly need to be done to confirm the extent of vinegar's benefits for type 2 diabetes patients and those at risk of developing this increasingly common disease. But for now, people with type 2 diabetes might be wise to talk with their doctors or dietitians about consuming more vinegar.

REPLACING UNHEALTHY FATS AND SODIUM

As you'll discover in chapter four, there are some delicious varieties of vinegar available. Each bestows a different taste or character to foods. The diversity and intensity of flavor are key to one important healing role that vinegar can play. Whether you are trying to protect yourself from cardiovascular diseases, such as heart disease, high blood pressure, or stroke, or you have been diagnosed with one or more of these conditions and have been advised to clean up your diet, vinegar should become a regular cooking and dining companion. That's because a tasty vinegar can often be used in place of sodium and/or ingredients high in saturated or *trans* fats to add flavor and excitement to a variety of dishes.

Saturated and *trans* fats have been shown to have a detrimental effect on blood cholesterol levels (see pages 110-111 for a more detailed discussion of the link between these fats and high blood cholesterol levels), and experts recommend that people who have or are at risk of developing high blood pressure cut back on the amount of sodium they consume. So using vinegar as a simple, flavorful substitute for these less healthful ingredients as often as possible can help people manage blood cholesterol and blood pressure levels and, in turn, help ward off heart disease and stroke.

You'll find detailed advice about including more vinegar in your diet in chapter four, and you'll discover delicious, good-for-you recipes at the end of the book that put vinegar to use. But the following suggestions will give you some sense of how vinegar can help you create and enjoy a diet that may lower your blood cholesterol and blood pressure and decrease your risks of heart disease and stroke:

♦ Make a vinegar-based coleslaw rather than a creamy, mayonnaise-based one. Because mayonnaise is made up almost completely of unhealthy fats and cholesterol, this easy switch can dramatically reduce the cholesterol and fat in this popular side dish.

♦ Enjoy healthier fish and chips. Instead of dipping fish in tartar sauce and drenching fries in salt and ketchup, splash them with a little malt vinegar. (Also consider baking the fish and the potatoes instead of frying them.) Because it contains mayonnaise, tartar sauce is high in unhealthy fats and cholesterol.

♦ Use vinegar-based salad dressings instead of creamy, mayonnaise-based dressings. Choose or make a flavorful herb salad dressing that contains mostly water, vinegar, and just a touch of oil to help it adhere to your salad veggies.

◆ Opt for vinegar instead of mayonnaise or other common, bad-fat-laden sandwich spreads to add flavor and moisture to sandwiches.

◆ When making a dish that contains beans, add a little vinegar near the end of cooking—it will dramatically decrease the amount of salt you'll need. It perks up the flavor of beans without raising your blood pressure.

◆ You can also use vinegar as a tangy marinade for tenderizing less-fatty cuts of meat. Choosing meat with less fat on the edges and less marbling within is one of the easiest ways to trim unhealthy fats from your diet. Unfortunately, meats that don't have as much marbling tend to be a little tougher. So vinegar can do double duty by adding a dash of zing as it tenderizes.

Making a Healthy Diet Easier to Swallow

Some of our strongest natural weapons against cancer and aging are fruits and vegetables. The antioxidants and phytochemicals they contain seem to hold real promise in lowering our risk of many types of cancer. Their antioxidants also help to protect cells from the free-radical damage that is thought to underlie many of the changes we associate with aging. Protected cells don't wear out and need replacing as often as cells that aren't bathed in antioxidants. Scientists think this continual cell replacement may be at the root of aging.

The U.S. government's 2005 Dietary Guidelines recommend that the average person eat about two cups of fruit and two-

ADD FLAVOR, NOT CALORIES

Vinegar contains very few calories—only 25 in half a cup! Compare that to the nearly 800 calories you get in half a cup of mayonnaise, and you have a real fat-fighting food. So if you're looking to lose weight, using vinegar in place of mayonnaise whenever you can will help you make a serious dent in your calorie (and fat) intake.

Vinegar can also help you have your dessert and cut calories, too. Use a splash of balsamic vinegar to bring out the sweetness and flavor of strawberries without any added sugar. Try it on other fruits that you might sprinkle sugar on—you'll be pleasantly surprised at the difference a bit of balsamic vinegar can make. And for a real unexpected treat on a hot summer evening, drizzle balsamic vinegar—instead of high-fat, sugary caramel or chocolate sauce—on a dish of reduced-fat vanilla ice cream. Can't imagine that combination? Just try it.

and-a-half cups of vegetables every day. One way to add excitement and variety to all those vegetables is to use vinegar liberally as a seasoning.

◆ Rice vinegar and a little soy sauce give veggies an Asian flavor or can form the base of an Asian coleslaw.

◆ Red wine vinegar or white wine vinegar can turn boring vegetables into a quick-and-easy marinated-vegetable salad that's ready to grab out of the refrigerator whenever hunger strikes. Just chop your favorite veggies, put them in a bowl with a marinade of vinegar, herbs, and a dash of olive oil, and let them sit for at least an hour. (You don't need much oil to make the marinade stick to the veggies, so go light, and be sure you choose olive oil.)

◆ Toss chopped vegetables in a vinegar-and-olive-oil salad dressing before loading them on skewers and putting them on the backyard grill. The aroma and flavor will actually have your family asking for seconds—*of vegetables!*

◆ After steaming vegetables, drizzle a little of your favorite vinegar over them instead of adding butter or salt. They'll taste so good, you may never get to the meat on your plate.

By enhancing the flavor of vegetables with vinegar, you and your family will be inclined to eat more of them. And that— many researchers and doctors would agree—will likely go a long way toward protecting your body's cells from the damage that can lead to cancer and other problems of aging.

REMOVING HARMFUL SUBSTANCES FROM PRODUCE

Some people are concerned that eating large amounts of fruits and vegetables may lead to an unhealthy consumption of pesticide and other farm-chemical residues. Vinegar can lend a hand here, too. Washing produce in a mixture of water and vinegar appears to help remove certain pesticides, according to the small amount of research that has been published. Vinegar also appears to be helpful in getting rid of harmful bacteria on fruits and vegetables.

To help remove potentially harmful residues, mix a solution of 10 percent vinegar to 90 percent water (for example, mix one cup of white vinegar in nine cups of water). Then, place produce in the vinegar solution, let it soak briefly, and then swish it around in the solution. Finally, rinse the produce thoroughly.

Do not use this process on tender, fragile fruits, such as berries, that might be damaged in the process or soak up too much vinegar through their porous skins.

Some pesticide residues are trapped beneath the waxy coatings that are applied to certain vegetables to help them retain moisture. The vinegar solution probably won't wash those pesticides away, so peeling lightly may be the next best option. Some research suggests that cooking further eliminates some pesticide residue.

THE SOUR THAT'S REALLY SWEET

Obviously, much more research needs to be done to investigate all of vinegar's healing potential. But even with the evidence available, it's clear that vinegar holds some healing powers. It is not a too-good-to-be-true miracle cure, but it can be used in a variety of ways to enhance your efforts to fight serious, chronic diseases (and as noted in the box on pages 75 and 76, it may lend a healing hand against some common, minor discomforts).

In that sense, vinegar is like many of the other lifestyle adjustments, drugs, and therapies used in our battles against common, chronic, and often life-threatening diseases: It is just one of a variety of important steps that can help us defend ourselves. But unlike many of the other elements that go into treating or preventing disease, vinegar is one you'll certainly enjoy incorporating into your life. In chapter four, you'll find the practical information you need to make vinegar a staple of your healing kitchen.

THE TRUTH ABOUT VINEGAR SUPPLEMENTS

Some people believe in the healing power of apple cider vinegar but would rather take it in tablet form instead of using it as a daily tonic or adding it to food. But like any shortcut on the road to better health, you can't be sure this one will get you to the goal you're aiming for.

Part of the reason for concern is that the U.S. Food and Drug Administration does not regulate supplements, so you really can't be sure what you're getting. In a study reported in the July 2005 *Journal of the American Dietetic Association,* for example, researchers analyzed eight different brands of apple cider vinegar tablets. The analysis showed most had acetic acid levels different from what was claimed on the label. How much of a problem is this? Well, it would be natural to think the more acetic acid the better. But in truth, at a level of 11 percent, acetic acid can cause burns to the skin. And at 20 percent, it is considered poisonous.

Some of the analyzed supplements, however, claimed to contain a frightening 35 percent acetic acid! Fortunately for their users, none did. The acetic acid content actually ranged from 1.04 percent to 10.57 percent. And another reason to go natural: Several of the samples were contaminated with mold and/or yeast, including one that claimed to be yeast-free.

In addition, because so little scientific research has been done to verify the healing claims made for vinegar—and the possible ingredients or actions that might be responsible—it's impossible to know if supplements would have the same actions and effects as the real thing. Indeed, most of the healing claims made for vinegar that seem to rest on the most solid scientific grounds are those based on vinegar's use as a substitute for unhealthy ingredients in the diet—a role that simply could not be played by a pill.

So at this time, it would seem you are almost certainly better off including more vinegar in your diet, taking advantage of its potential healing benefits as well as its phenomenal flavors, rather than spending more money on supplements that may not have any benefit and could even be dangerous.

CHAPTER FOUR
VINEGAR IN THE KITCHEN

With a splash here or a half-cup there, vinegar adds zing and zest to your cooking and brings out the flavors of other foods. No kitchen pantry is complete without at least a few different types of this flavor-enhancer. Vinegar is a must-have ingredient for vinaigrettes, marinades, food preservation, or any recipe that needs a little extra kick.

You might be surprised to learn that there are dozens of types of vinegar. The most common vinegars found in American kitchens are white distilled and apple cider, but the more adventurous may also use red wine vinegar; white wine vinegar; rice vinegar; or gourmet varieties, such as 25-year-old balsamic vinegar or rich black fig vinegar.

As you've learned, vinegar can be made from just about any food that contains natural sugars. Yeast ferments these sugars into alcohol, and certain types of bacteria convert that alcohol a second time into vinegar. A weak acetic acid remains after this second fermentation; the acid has flavors reminiscent of the original fermented food, such as apples or grapes. Acetic acid is what gives vinegar its distinct tart taste.

Pure acetic acid can be made in a laboratory; when diluted with water, it is sometimes sold as white vinegar. However, acetic acids created in labs lack the subtle flavors found in true vinegars, and synthesized versions don't hold a candle to vinegars fermented naturally from summer's sugar-laden fruits or other foods.

Vinegars can be made from many different foods that add their own tastes to the final products, but additional ingredients, such as herbs, spices, or fruits, can be added for further flavor enhancement.

VINEGAR VARIETIES

Vinegar is great for a healthy, light style of cooking. The tangy taste often reduces the need for salt, especially in soups and bean dishes. It can also cut the fat in a recipe because it balances flavors without requiring the addition of as much cream, butter, or oil. Vinegar flavors range from mild to bold, so you're sure to find one with the taste you want. A brief look at some of the various vinegars available may help you choose a new one for your culinary escapades.

WHITE VINEGAR

This clear variety is the most common type of vinegar in American households. It is made either from grain-based ethanol or laboratory-produced acetic acid and then diluted with water. Its flavor is a bit too harsh for most cooking uses, but it is good for pickling and performing many cleaning jobs around the house.

APPLE CIDER VINEGAR

Apple cider vinegar is the second-most-common type of vinegar in the United States. This light-tan vinegar made from apple cider adds a tart and subtle fruity flavor to your cooking. Apple cider vinegar is best for salads, dressings, marinades, condiments, and most general vinegar needs.

PASTEURIZED FOR YOUR PROTECTION

Some apple cider vinegars proudly proclaim to be "raw, organic, and unpasteurized," but beware: Buying an unpasteurized product is risky business.

Most apple cider is made from apples that have fallen to the ground, and the bacterium *E. coli* can easily contaminate these fruits. If processors don't wash off this deadly bacterium before the apples are pressed, and the final product is not pasteurized, there is a risk of *E. coli* contamination, which can lead to severe health problems and even death. Although most bacteria cannot survive in the acidic conditions of vinegar, the acidity of the unpasteurized product can weaken over time, thus allowing bacteria to grow—and making the product dangerous for you.

To be on the safe side, be sure you always choose vinegars that have been prepared, pasteurized, and stored properly.

WINE VINEGAR

This flavorful type of vinegar is made from a blend of either red wines or white wines and is common in Europe, especially Germany. Creative cooks often infuse wine vinegars with extra flavor by tucking in a few sprigs of well-washed fresh herbs, dried herbs, or fresh berries. Red wine vinegar is often flavored with natural raspberry flavoring, if not with the fruit itself.

The quality of the original wine determines how good the vinegar is. Better wine vinegars are made from good wines and are aged for a couple of years or more in wooden casks. The result is a fuller, more complex, and mellow flavor.

You might find sherry vinegar on the shelf next to the wine vinegars. This variety is made from sherry wine, and usually is imported from Spain. Champagne vinegar (yes, made from the bubbly stuff) is a specialty vinegar and is quite expensive.

Wine vinegar excels at bringing out the sweetness of fruit, melon, and berries and adds a flavorful punch to fresh salsa.

BALSAMIC VINEGAR

There are two types of this popular and flavorful vinegar, traditional and commercial. A quasigovernmental body in Modena, Italy (balsamic vinegar's birthplace), regulates the production of traditional balsamic vinegar.

Traditional balsamic. Traditional balsamic vinegars are artisanal foods, similar to great wines, with long histories and well-developed customs for their production. An excellent balsamic vinegar can be made only by an experienced crafter who has spent many years tending the vinegar, patiently watching and learning.

The luscious white and sugary trebbiano grapes that are grown in the northern region of Italy near Modena form the base of the world's best and only true balsamic vinegars. Customdictates that the grapes be left on the vine for as long as possible to develop their sugar. The juice (or "must") is pressed out of the grapes and boiled down; then, vinegar production begins.

A TRIO OF FUNCTIONS

Vinegar is an invaluable kitchen staple that can be put to use in three important ways:

- It provides seasoning and a flavor boost.

- It acts as a preservative that can turn cucumbers and other summer vegetables into delicious pickles that can be safely stored for later use.

- It is useful in marinades to tenderize tough meat.

Traditional balsamic vinegar is aged for a number of years— typically 6 and as many as 25. Aging takes place in a succession of casks made from a variety of woods, such as chestnut, mulberry, oak, juniper, and cherry. Each producer has its own formula for the order in which the vinegar is moved to the different casks. Thus, the flavors are complex, rich, sweet, and subtly woody. Vinegar made in this way carries a seal from the Consortium of Producers of the Traditional Balsamic Vinegar of Modena.

Because of the arduous production process, only a limited amount of traditional balsamic vinegar makes it to market each year, and what is available is expensive.

Leaf ratings. You might see that some traditional balsamic vinegars have leaves on their labels. This is a rating system that ranks quality on a one- to four-leaf scale, with four leaves being the best. You can use the leaf ranking as a guide for how to use the vinegar. For instance, one-leaf balsamic vinegar would be appropriate for salad dressing, while four-leaf vinegar would be best used a few drops at a time to season a dish right before serving. The Assaggiatori Italiani Balsamico (Italian Balsamic Tasters' Association) established this grading system, but not all producers use it.

Commercial balsamic. What you're more likely to find in most American grocery stores is the commercial type of balsamic vinegar. Some is made in Modena, but not by traditional methods. In fact, some balsamic vinegar isn't even made in Italy. Commercial balsamic vinegar does not carry the Consortium of Producers of the Traditional Balsamic Vinegar of Modena seal because it is not produced in accordance with the Consortium's strict regulations.

The production of commercial balsamic vinegar carries no geographical restrictions or rules for length or method of aging. There are no requirements for the types of wood used in the aging casks. It may be aged for six months in stainless steel vats, then for two years or more in wood. Thus, commercial balsamic vinegar is much more affordable and available than the true, artisanal variety.

Whether you're lucky enough to get your hands on the traditional variety or you're using commercial-grade balsamic, the taste of this fine vinegar is like no other. Its sweet and sour notes are in perfect proportion. Balsamic's flavor is so intricate that it brings out the best in salty foods such as goat cheese, astringent foods such as spinach, and sweet foods such as strawberries.

RICE VINEGAR

Clear or very pale yellow, rice vinegar originated in Japan, where it is essential to sushi preparation. Rice vinegar is made from the sugars found in rice, and the aged, filtered final product has a mild, clean, and delicate flavor that is an excellent complement to ginger or cloves, sometimes with the addition of sugar.

Rice vinegar also comes in red and black varieties, which are less common in the United States but very popular in China. Both are stronger than the clear (often called white) or pale yellow types. Red rice vinegar's flavor is a combination of sweet and tart. Black rice vinegar is common in southern Chinese cooking and has a strong, almost smoky flavor.

Rice vinegar is popular in Asian cooking and is great sprinkled on salads and stir-fry dishes. Its gentle flavor is perfect for fruits and tender vegetables, too. Many cooks choose white rice vinegar for their recipes because it does not change the color of the food to which it is added. Red rice vinegar is good for soups and noodle dishes, and black rice vinegar works as a dipping sauce and in braised dishes.

Malt Vinegar

This dark-brown vinegar, a favorite in Britain, is reminiscent of deep-brown ale. Malt vinegar production begins with the germination, or sprouting, of barley kernels. Germination enables enzymes to break down starch. Sugar is formed, and the resulting product is brewed into an alcohol-containing malt beverage or ale. After bacteria convert the ale to vinegar, the vinegar is aged. As its name implies, malt vinegar has a distinctive malt flavor.

Last-Minute Splash

Vinegar loses some of its pungency when heated. If you want to enjoy vinegar's full tart taste, add it to a dish at the end of cooking. Also, after heating up leftovers, splash them with vinegar to perk up their flavors.

A cheaper and less flavorful version of malt vinegar consists merely of acetic acid diluted to between 4 percent and 8 percent acidity with a little caramel coloring added.

Many people prefer malt vinegar for pickling and as an accompaniment to fish and chips. It is also used as the basic type of cooking vinegar in Britain.

Cane Vinegar

This type of vinegar is produced from the sugar cane and is used mainly in the Philippines. It is often light yellow and has a flavor similar to rice vinegar. Contrary to what you might think, cane vinegar is not any sweeter than other vinegars.

BEER VINEGAR

Beer vinegar has an appealing light-golden color and, as you might guess, is popular in Germany, Austria, Bavaria, and the Netherlands. It is made from beer, and its flavor depends on the brew from which it was made. It has a sharp, malty taste.

COCONUT VINEGAR

If you can't get your Asian recipes to taste "just right," it might be because you don't have coconut vinegar—a white vinegar with a sharp, acidic, slightly yeasty taste. This staple of Southeast Asian cooking is made from the sap of the coconut palm and is especially important to Thai and Indian dishes.

RAISIN VINEGAR

This slightly cloudy brown vinegar is traditionally produced in Turkey and used in Middle Eastern cuisines. Try infusing it with a little cinnamon to bolster its mild flavor. Salad dressings made with raisin vinegar will add an unconventional taste to your greens.

MAKE YOUR OWN APPLE CIDER VINEGAR

Perhaps reading about all these exciting kinds of vinegar has whetted your appetite to make some of your own. Experimenting with flavors can be fun, and it's especially rewarding when you use your own vinegar in favorite dishes or give it as a gift.

You'll want to get exact directions from your local brewing supply store or university extension service. Be sure the

ALL ABOUT ACIDITY

The U.S. Food and Drug Administration requires that vinegar contain a minimum of 4 percent acetic acid. White vinegar is typically 5 percent acetic acid, and cider and wine vinegars are a bit more acidic, usually between 5 percent and 6 percent.

A little acidity goes a long way—acetic acid is corrosive and can destroy living tissues when concentrated. An acetic acid level of 11 percent or more can burn the skin. And according to the Consumer Product Safety Commission, an "acetic acid preparation containing free or chemically unneutralized acetic acid in a concentration of 20 percent or more" is considered poison. In fact, a 20 percent acetic acid concentration is sometimes used as an herbicide to kill garden weeds.

directions you follow are tested and researched for safety to avoid food-borne illness. Take a look at this rundown of the general process to make apple cider vinegar to see if you're up to the task:

◆ Make apple cider by pressing clean, washed, ripe apples (fall apples have more sugar than early-season apples). Strain to make a clean juice and pour it into sterilized containers.

◆ Use yeast designed for brewing wine or beer (not baker's yeast) to ferment the fruit sugar into alcohol.

◆ Now let bacteria convert the alcohol to acetic acid. Leaving the fermenting liquid uncovered invites acid-making

MOTHER OF VINEGAR

If you see a jellylike cloudy film collecting in the bottom of your vinegar bottle, you've discovered the "mother of vinegar." It's merely cellulose made by acid-producing bacteria. Mother of vinegar is a completely natural by-product of vinegar that contains live bacteria. It is harmless and is not a sign of contamination. Just strain off the liquid vinegar and continue using it.

Most manufacturers pasteurize their vinegar to prevent the mother of vinegar from forming. Some say this goo prevents infectious diseases if you eat a little each day, but there is no research to verify that belief.

bacteria to take up residence (you might, however, want to place some cheesecloth or a towel over your container's opening to prevent insects, dirt, or other nasty items from getting into the mixture). Some vinegar brewers use a "mother of vinegar" (see box, above) as a "starter," or source of the acid-producing bacteria.

◆ Keep the liquid between 60 degrees and 80 degrees Fahrenheit during the fermentation process; it will take three to four weeks to make vinegar. If you keep the liquid too cool, the vinegar may be unusable. If it's kept too warm, it may not form the mother of vinegar mat at the bottom of the container. The mother of vinegar mat signifies proper fermentation. Stir the liquid daily to introduce adequate amounts of oxygen, which is necessary for fermentation.

- After three to four weeks, the bacteria will have converted most of the alcohol, and the mixture will begin to smell like vinegar. Taste a little bit each day until it reaches a flavor and acidity that you like.

- Strain the liquid through a cheesecloth or coffee filter several times to remove the mother of vinegar. Otherwise the fermentation process will continue and eventually spoil your vinegar.

- Store in sterilized, capped jars in the refrigerator.

- If you want to store homemade vinegar at room temperature for more than a few months, you must pasteurize it. Do this by heating it to 170 degrees Fahrenheit (use a cooking thermometer to determine the temperature) and hold it at this temperature for 10 minutes. Put the pasteurized vinegar in sterilized containers with tight-fitting lids, out of direct sunlight.

You can also make vinegar from wine; the process is similar.

FLAVOR INFUSION

Whether you start with homemade or store-bought vinegar, you can kick it up by adding flavorful herbs or spices. Garlic, basil, rosemary, and tarragon are herbs commonly added to white wine vinegar. Other herbs or fruits, such as raspberries, also can enhance vinegar's taste. These additions leave their flavors and trace amounts of healthy nutrients, too.

Herbal vinegars need to be carefully prepared to avoid contamination with potentially harmful bacteria. Most bacteria cannot exist in vinegar's acidic environment, but a few deadly ones can, so follow a few basic steps:

- Use only high-quality vinegars when creating flavor combinations. Typically, white wine vinegar or red wine vinegar are best for flavoring. Remember, though, that these vinegars contain trace amounts of protein that could give harmful bacteria an ideal place to live unless you prepare and store the vinegars properly.

- Wash your storage bottles and then sterilize them by completely immersing them in boiling water for ten minutes. Always fill the bottles while they are still warm, and be sure you have a tight-fitting lid, cap, or cork for each one.

- If you're using fresh herbs, there is a risk of harmful bacteria hitchhiking their way into the vinegar via the sprigs. Commercial vinegar processors use antimicrobial agents to sanitize herbs, but you probably won't be able to find these

A HOMEMADE-VINEGAR CAUTION

The acidity of homemade vinegar varies greatly. If you make your own vinegar, *do not* use it for canning, for preserving, or for anything that will be stored at room temperature. The vinegar's acidity, or pH level, may not be sufficient to preserve your food and could result in severe food poisoning. The pH level in homemade vinegar can weaken and allow pathogens, such as the deadly *E. coli*, to grow. Homemade vinegar is well suited for dressings, marinades, cooking, or pickled products that are stored in the refrigerator at all times.

chemicals. University extension publications recommend mixing one teaspoon of bleach into six cups of water and dipping the fresh herbs into this solution. Then rinse the herbs thoroughly and pat them dry. This will minimize the possibility of any harmful bacteria making their way into the vinegar and will not affect the taste.

◆ Be sure your fresh herbs are in top-notch condition—bruising or decay indicates the presence of bacteria. If you harvest your own herbs, do so in the morning, when the essential oils are at their peak. Use three to four sprigs or three tablespoons of dried herbs per pint of vinegar. Mix it up a bit by adding some spices or vegetables, such as garlic or hot peppers. Thread garlic, peppers, or other small items on a skewer so you can remove them easily when you've infused enough flavors.

◆ To add fruit flavors to vinegar, thoroughly wash fruit, berries, or citrus rind. Use one to two cups of fruit for every pint of vinegar, but only the rind of one lemon or orange per pint. You can thread small fruits or chunks of fruit on a skewer and tie chopped rind in a small piece of clean cheesecloth to make removal easy.

◆ When you're ready to start mixing, place the herbs or flavoring in the sterilized, hot bottles. Heat the vinegar to 190 degrees Fahrenheit and then pour it over the herbs in the sterilized bottles. Heating the vinegar to 190 degrees Fahrenheit will prevent bacteria from forming and also help release the essential oils from the herbs, spices, or fruits.

◆ Put a tight-fitting lid on your container and allow the vinegar to stand in a cool, dark place for three to four weeks. When it has enough flavor, strain it through a cheesecloth or coffee filter several times until any cloudiness is gone.

- Discard the fruits, spices, or herbs and pour the filtered vinegar into newly sterilized containers. If you want to add a decorative herb sprig, sanitize it using the method described earlier. Seal tightly.

- Store the vinegar in the refrigerator for the best flavor retention; it will keep well for six to eight months. Unrefrigerated vinegar will keep its flavor for only two to three months. If left to look pretty on a sunny windowsill for more than a few weeks, use the vinegar only as decoration, not as food.

- You can use your herbal vinegar in nearly any recipe that calls for plain vinegar.

THE BETTER OF TWO WORLDS

Vinegar is good for you, and garlic is great. Why not combine the two and make pickled garlic? Simply peel some garlic cloves, cube them, and let them sit for 10 to 15 minutes to form the allicin discussed in previous chapters. Then add the garlic to your favorite vinegar.

Vinegar helps garlic form healthful sulfur-containing compounds that are not otherwise formed in large amounts. The longer the garlic is in the vinegar, the more sulfur compounds it forms. Store your pickled garlic in the refrigerator and add it to salads and vegetable side dishes. What a delicious way to take your medicine— maybe a pickled clove a day will keep the doctor away.

Vinegar Magic

Storing vinegar properly will hold flavor at its peak. Due to their high acid content, commercially prepared vinegars will keep almost indefinitely, even at room temperature. White vinegar will maintain its color, but other kinds may develop an off color or a haze. Neither of these conditions is a sign of spoilage; the vinegar is still good to use.

Store all vinegars in bottles sealed with airtight lids. Keep in a dark, cool place, and avoid direct sunlight, which can diminish flavor, color, and acidity. Homemade vinegars, especially herbal ones, are best stored in the refrigerator.

Vinegar's acidity makes it a natural wonder in your kitchen. Besides the burst of flavor vinegar lends to whatever it touches, it serves other purposes, too:

◆ *Meat tenderizer:* Vinegar's acid helps break down muscle fibers in tough meats. Make a mixture of half vinegar and half broth, and soak tough meat in this solution for up to two hours. (Because of vinegar's ability to tenderize, never leave fish in a marinade that contains vinegar for longer than 20 minutes; otherwise the fish might get mushy.)

◆ *Fish poacher:* When poaching fish, put a tablespoon of vinegar in the poaching water to keep the fish from falling apart. Vinegar helps the protein in the fish coagulate, and mushiness isn't a problem because fish is usually poached for less than 20 minutes.

◆ *Egg saver:* Put a tablespoon of vinegar in the water when boiling eggs. If any eggs crack while dancing in the water, their whites will coagulate and not escape from the shells.

◆ **Buttermilk stand-in:** When a recipe calls for buttermilk and you have none, substitute plain milk and add a little vinegar. Use one tablespoon of vinegar per cup (eight ounces) of milk. Let stand 10 to 15 minutes at room temperature until it thickens, then use it in your recipe as you would buttermilk. Choose mild-flavored vinegar, such as apple cider vinegar, for this purpose.

◆ *Candy smoother:* When making homemade candy and icing, a few drops of vinegar will prevent the texture from getting grainy.

◆ *Potato whitener:* Cover peeled potatoes with water and a tablespoon or two of vinegar to keep them from browning.

◆ *Food preserver:* Use vinegar to make pickles or to can vegetables to preserve the freshness of your garden or local farm stand. The U.S. Department of Agriculture (USDA) publishes up-to-date information about pickling, canning, and preserving. These instructions will yield tasty pickles and home-canned products that are safe to eat. Check your local state university extension office or the USDA Web site (www.usda.gov) for tips about pickling.

VINEGAR'S VIM

No matter how you look at it, vinegar can add spice to your culinary life. Prowl the gourmet shops in your area and you'll find dozens of different vinegars. Select a few to bring home and put them to use with the recipes in this book. Your taste buds will definitely be pleased, but it may be your health that benefits most.

VINEGAR TO THE RESCUE!

Let vinegar solve some common, frustrating household problems:

- Pour about a teaspoon of vinegar into a nearly empty mayonnaise jar and swish it around to get out the last of the mayonnaise.

- Use it to remove berry stains from your hands.

- Soak a paper towel with vinegar and place it in a smelly lunchbox overnight to remove those hard-to-get-rid-of odors.

- Simmer a small saucepan of water and vinegar to remove cooking smells from the kitchen.

- Add vinegar to a piecrust recipe and the dough will be easier to roll out. (The crust may be less flaky, however.) Most recipes call for about a tablespoon of vinegar for a double crust.

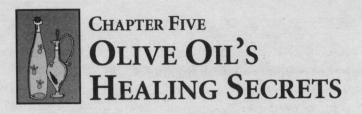

CHAPTER FIVE
OLIVE OIL'S HEALING SECRETS

Olive oil completes our triumvirate of nature's healing wonders. This liquid gold works to keep hearts healthy, may reduce inflammation and the risk of certain cancers, and might even play a role in controlling diabetes and weight.

A diet that is rich in olive oil has enhanced the health of people living in the Mediterranean region for thousands of years. Within the past century, however, olive oil's benefits have also been scientifically investigated, acknowledged, and proclaimed across the globe.

Many theories exist as to where olive trees originated, but one that is fairly well accepted is that they first grew in Asia Minor, the land bridge between Europe and Asia that is now home to Turkey and Syria. Evidence shows that humans in this area were using olives more than 8,000 years ago.

Historians believe olive use spread throughout the rest of the Mediterranean region about 6,000 years ago. Phoenicians carried olive trees to what is now southern Europe, as well as to Egypt and other areas along the North African coast. Like garlic, olive remnants have been found inside Egyptian tombs, signifying the important role they played in that culture.

THE HARDY OLIVE TREE

An olive tree can live 1,000 years or more. Even if the tree dies or is cut or damaged, sprouts from its roots can grow into full-size, fruit-bearing trees. Olive trees succeed in climates in which there are mildly cold winters (they need cooler temperatures to set the buds that later form the fruit) and long, hot summers. During the growing season, olives need a lot of dry heat. The tough trees don't need much water and can tolerate temperatures as low as 10 degrees Fahrenheit for brief periods of time.

Later, the Greeks and Romans put olives to good use. People in both of these ancient civilizations used olive oil to counteract poisons and to treat open wounds, insect bites, headaches, and stomach and digestive problems. They also applied olive oil to the body before bathing (it functioned as soap) and then again afterward to moisturize the skin and to form a barrier against dirt and the sun's rays. The Romans took olives along in their travels, planting them wherever they went and spreading their beneficial qualities to many regions.

HEALING THROUGH THE AGES

The olive's medicinal properties have helped people for thousands of years, and those who reaped the benefits of the fruit didn't keep its wonderful secrets to themselves. During the past several hundred years, olive trees made their way around the world to areas in which they could be successfully cultivated, including North America, South America, New Zealand, Australia, and Japan.

As the olive migrated, folk remedies that used olive oil evolved to reflect the times and maladies of different regions. Olive oil was taken by mouth, spread on the skin, and dropped into the ears or nose. People considered it both a cure and a preventative measure for many afflictions. Here are some popular folk remedies that have been used over the years:

♦ Take a spoonful or two to treat an upset stomach, difficult digestion, or constipation or to reduce the body's absorption of alcohol from alcoholic beverages.

♦ Apply to skin to prevent dryness and wrinkles, to soften the skin, and to treat acne.

♦ Use on the hair to make it shiny and to treat dandruff.

♦ Strengthen nails by soaking them in warm olive oil.

♦ Ease aching muscles by massaging them with olive oil.

♦ Lower blood pressure by boiling olive tree leaves and drinking the "tea."

♦ Clear nasal congestion with drops of olive oil in the nose.

A word of caution: Using olive oil as a folk remedy may not be safe for children. In November 2005, an article in *Archives of Pediatrics & Adolescent Medicine* and an ensuing report by Reuters Health cautioned caregivers against giving infants and young children a dose of olive oil to treat digestive problems, fussiness, and stuffy noses. Oil administered through the mouth or nose may be inhaled into the lungs and can cause lipoid pneumonia. You should always consult a pediatrician before trying any treatment—whether folk remedy or over-the-counter drug—on a child.

A GOD'S GIFT

According to Greek mythology, Athena, daughter of Zeus, invented the olive tree and gave it to the people of Athens as a gift. As the story goes, Athena planted the first olive tree on a hill now known as the Acropolis. Some say the olive tree that grows there today comes from the roots of that original tree. The Greeks appreciated the olive so much that they named their capital city after the goddess who gave them the tree.

Chronic diseases and conditions that are caused, in part, by unhealthy foods and sedentary lifestyles plague many societies today, especially those in the Western world. The good news is olive oil may help with the worst of them, including heart disease, hypertension (high blood pressure), metabolic syndrome, inflammation, cancer, diabetes, and problems associated with obesity.

These conditions take many years to develop, but inactivity and consumption of too much solid fat (saturated fat and *trans* fat) greatly increase your chances of having to deal with them. However, olive oil and diets rich in monounsaturated fat may help combat the development of some chronic conditions.

FAT FACTS

It may seem remarkable that such a small dietary change— switching from one type of fat to another—can significantly impact your health, but as you will see here, the type of fat you fancy really matters. Some fats, especially olive oil, have more healthful properties than others, so to make the right choices, it's important to know the differences among the various kinds.

There are four types of dietary fats, also known as fatty acids, and each has different health effects, depending on its source and how it is produced.

Monounsaturated fat. This is the healthiest type of fat. It promotes heart health and might help prevent cancer and a host of other ailments. Monounsaturated fat helps lower "bad" LDL cholesterol levels without negatively affecting the "good" HDL cholesterol (see pages 17-18 for more about the differences between LDL and HDL cholesterol). Olive oil, peanut oil, canola oil, and avocados are rich in healthy monounsaturated fat.

Polyunsaturated fat. Polyunsaturated fat is moderately healthy. It lowers LDL cholesterol, which is good, but it also reduces levels of artery-clearing HDL cholesterol. Polyunsaturated fat is usually liquid at room temperature and is the predominant type of fatty acid in soybean oil, safflower oil, corn oil, and several other vegetable oils.

Saturated fat. This fat is unhealthy because the body turns it into artery-clogging cholesterol, which is harmful to your heart. Saturated fat is mostly found in animal products and is solid at room temperature. It is the white fat you see along the edge or marbled throughout a piece of meat and is the fat in the skin of poultry. It is also "hidden" in whole milk and foods made from whole milk, as well as in tropical oils such as coconut oil. Dietitians recommend that people eat only small amounts of saturated fat.

Trans *fat*. *Trans* fat is the worst type of fat; you're best off avoiding it. Most *trans* fat is manufactured by forcing hydrogen into liquid polyunsaturated fat in a process called hydrogenation. The process can create a solid fat product—margarine is made this way. Hydrogenation gives foods that contain *trans* fats a longer shelf life and helps stabilize their flavors, but your body pays a big price.

The body recognizes *trans* fat as being saturated and converts it to cholesterol, which raises LDL levels and lowers HDL levels. What's worse is that unlike saturated fat, *trans* fat disrupts cell membranes. Cell membranes are comprised of uniformly configured fatty acid chains that are linked together through tight chemical bonds. When *trans* fat works its way into the chains, it alters these bonds and creates "leaks" in the cell membrane. This action upsets the flow of nutrients and waste products into and out of the cell and may be linked to reduced immune function and possibly cancer.

Fried foods in restaurants may contain large amounts of *trans* fats if they are cooked in partially hydrogenated oil. However, thanks to pressure from consumer and health groups, some restaurants are now using liquid soybean oil rather than partially hydrogenated soybean oil. This costs the restaurant a little more but is healthier for you.

Many fast-food restaurant chains display a nutrition facts brochure—check this literature to see how much *trans* fat is in each food. When dining elsewhere, ask your server whether the cooks use a *trans*-fat-free oil. When frying foods at home, be

YOUR RIGHT TO KNOW

By rule of the United States Food and Drug Administration (FDA), as of January 1, 2006, food manufacturers are required to list the amount of *trans* fat on nutrition labels. The FDA rule states that the amount of *trans* fat in a serving should be listed by weight (in grams) on a separate line under saturated fat.

However, according to the FDA, food manufacturers are allowed to list the amount of *trans* fat per serving in a food as zero grams if the actual amount is less than 0.5 gram. That is why you may see a product that has partially hydrogenated vegetable oil listed as an ingredient but has *trans* fat content listed as zero grams.

sure to use a liquid oil, such as heart-healthy olive oil, rather than shortening, which is created by hydrogenation.

Meat and milk are also sources of *trans* fat, but they contain very little. These naturally occurring *trans* fats do not appear to have any negative health consequences.

MAJORITY RULES

The fat we eat is made up of varying amounts of the different fats just described. When a food is predominantly comprised of one type of fat, we call it by that name. For instance, as the chart on the next page shows, olive oil is high in monounsaturated fat. Even though it contains other types of fat, olive oil is referred to as a monounsaturated fat. You'll see at a glance that olive oil outweighs any other fat when it comes to health-promoting monounsaturated fat content.

Type of fat	% monounsat- urated fat	% poly- unsaturated fat	% saturated fat	% other elements
Olive oil	74	8	14	4
Canola oil	59	30	7	4
Peanut oil	46	32	17	5
Corn oil	24	59	13	4
Soybean oil	23	58	14	4
Sunflower oil	20	65	10	5
Safflower oil	14	75	6	5
Walnut oil	23	63	9	5
Palm kernel oil	11	2	81	6
Palm oil	37	9	50	4
Coconut oil	6	2	86	6
Butter	30	4	62	4
Shortening	30	37	29	4
*Tallow	42	4	50	4

*Rendered fat of cattle or sheep

Note: Due to rounding, not all values will equal 100 percent for each type of fat

Source: U.S. Department of Agriculture, Agricultural Research Service. 2005. USDA National Nutrient Database for Standard Reference, Release 18. Nutrient Data Laboratory Home Page, www.ars.usda.gov/ba/bhnrc/ndl

An Olive's Omegas

There are two important polyunsaturated fats that are essential for human health, but the body cannot make them. This means we must get them from the foods we eat. These two essential fatty acids are alpha-linolenic acid, an omega-3 fatty acid, and linoleic acid, an omega-6 fatty acid. The body gets both from olive oil.

Omega-3 oils are the healthiest. They are part of a group of substances called prostaglandins that help keep blood cells from sticking together, increase blood flow, and reduce inflammation. This makes omega-3 oils useful in preventing cardiovascular disease as well as inflammatory conditions, such as arthritis.

Omega-6 oils are healthy, too, but they are not quite as helpful as omega-3's. Omega-6's can help form prostaglandins that are similarly beneficial to the ones produced by omega-3's, but they can also produce harmful prostaglandins. The unfavorable prostaglandins increase blood-cell stickiness and promote cardiovascular disease, and they also appear to be linked to the formation of cancer. To encourage your body to make beneficial prostaglandins from omega-6 oils, you should decrease the amount of animal fats you eat. Too many animal fats tend to push your body into using omega-6 oils to make the unfavorable prostaglandins rather than the helpful ones.

The research is inconclusive about how much omega-6 you should eat compared to the amount of omega-3. Many researchers suggest consuming one to four times more omega-6's than omega-3's. However, the typical American eats anywhere from 11 to 30 times more omega-6's than omega-3's.

The U.S. Dietary Reference Intakes for essential fatty acids recommends the consumption of omega-6 and omega-3 fats in a ratio of 10-to-1. This means consuming ten times more omega-6's than omega-3's. Lucky for us, nature provided that exact ratio of fat in each little olive. The linoleic-to-linolenic ratio is about 10-to-1.

GET HEART HELP FROM OLIVE OIL

Research abounds regarding the benefits of monounsaturated fat. Other studies are showing that the potent phytochemicals (those substances in plants that may have health benefits for people) in olive oil—specifically, a group called phenolic compounds—appear to promote good health.

Studies have shown that a phytochemical in olive oil called hydroxytyrosol "thins" the blood. Other phytochemicals reduce inflammation of the blood vessels, prevent oxidation of fats in the bloodstream, protect blood vessel walls, and dilate the blood vessels for improved circulation.

CHOLESTEROL COMBATANT

Olive oil boosts heart health by keeping a lid on cholesterol levels. It lowers total cholesterol, LDL cholesterol, and triglyceride levels. Some studies show that it does not affect HDL cholesterol; others show that it slightly increases HDL levels.

A 2002 article in *The American Journal of Medicine* reported that total cholesterol levels decrease an average of 13.4 percent

JUICE VS. SEEDS

Olives are a fruit, and when you press them, you get juice. This juice is rich not only in oil but also in potent phytochemicals and several vitamins. Need another reason to choose olive oil? It's a more natural product than seed oils.

Seeds, such as sunflower, soybean, or rapeseed (the source of canola oil), undergo much more processing to extract their oil. They are not merely crushed or pressed to remove their oil; they are typically processed with heat and sometimes chemicals to gain access to their tiny oil reserves. Even "cold-pressed" seed oils require heat of up to 120 degrees Fahrenheit. Therefore, seed oil is more highly processed than what we get from simple olive juice.

and LDL cholesterol levels drop an average of 18 percent when people replace saturated fat with monounsaturated fat in their diets. These results seem to hold for middle-age and older adults who have high blood cholesterol levels.

The polyphenolic compounds (types of phytochemicals) in olive oil appear to play a big part in protecting blood vessels. Three polyphenols, oleuropein, tyrosol, and hydroxytyrosol, are believed to be particularly helpful. Numerous studies have shown that polyphenols and monounsaturated fat help keep LDL cholesterol from being oxidized and getting stuck to the inner walls of arteries, which forms the plaque that hampers blood flow. When plaque forms in arteries, the risk of heart disease or stroke increases.

Polyphenolic compounds are also responsible for preserving and protecting two enzymes—glutathione reductase and glutathione peroxidase—that fight free radicals in the body. Without enzymes like these, free radicals can damage healthy cells, potentially leading to the development of cancer and other serious health problems.

NOW READ THIS!

The FDA approved a health claim statement in November 2004 for optional use on labels of foods that are rich in monounsaturated fat and low in cholesterol and saturated fat. It reads:

"Limited and not conclusive scientific evidence suggests that eating about 2 tablespoons (23 grams) of olive oil daily may reduce the risk of coronary heart disease due to the monounsaturated fat in olive oil. To achieve this possible benefit, olive oil is to replace a similar amount of saturated fat and not increase the total number of calories you eat in a day. One serving of this product contains [x] grams of olive oil."

The last sentence is optional when the claim is used on actual olive oil labels.

Research reported in the November 2005 issue of the *Journal of the American College of Cardiology* provides compelling evidence for the advantages of olive oil's polyphenolic compounds. In the study, 21 otherwise-healthy Spanish volunteers who had high blood cholesterol levels were given 2.5 tablespoons of either virgin olive oil that was rich in phenolic compounds or olive oil that had much less of these phytonutrients as part of their breakfast. Careful measurements for the next four hours showed that those who consumed the phenolic-rich olive oil experienced:

◆ An increase in the dilation of the interior walls of blood vessels. The more dilated a vessel is, the freer the circulation and the less work the heart has to do to pump blood through the body.

◆ An increase in the amount of nitric oxide in the bloodstream. Nitric oxide is a strong vasodilator (an agent that causes the blood vessels to dilate, or expand). Nitric oxide relaxes the smooth muscles that line artery walls, thus improving circulation. It also inhibits the clumping of blood cells called platelets, reducing the risk of blood clots. Oleuropein is the phytonutrient in olive oil that is responsible for stimulating the production of nitric oxide.

Results such as these suggest that adding a small amount of phenolic-rich olive oil to the diet (or, better yet, substituting olive oil for harmful saturated fats in the diet) can make a significant impact on reducing atherosclerosis and the cascade of events that lead to heart disease. The researchers identified this finding as especially important because, in other studies, meals high in saturated fat, such as hamburgers and french fries, have been shown to create the opposite effect. Such meals

GET TO KNOW NITRIC OXIDE

In the environment, nitric oxide is a by-product of our love affair with the automobile. It's expelled as part of a car's exhaust and contributes to the smog that hangs over our urban areas. So it's surprising that in the body, nitric oxide is a good thing. For example, it improves blood flow by relaxing the smooth muscles that line blood vessel walls, thinning the blood and decreasing inflammation in blood vessels. The medication nitroglycerine actually creates nitric oxide in the body to treat angina. With this condition, the myocardium (the thick, muscular middle layer of the heart wall) doesn't get enough oxygen, usually because blood vessels are obstructed. This causes great pain in the chest and arms. Nitroglycerine creates nitric oxide that helps blood vessels relax. When this happens, circulation increases, and pain subsides.

Improved blood flow also helps prevent hypertension, increases kidney function, and enhances penile erections in men. It also relaxes other muscles so they get more oxygen and don't cramp. Intestines depend on nitric oxide for peristalsis, which is the wavelike motion that moves food through your digestive system. And certain immune cells produce nitric oxide to fight bacteria.

inhibit the normal and healthy function of blood vessels and constrict blood flow.

Taking the two sets of results together, then, further enhances support for the cardiac benefits of using olive oil in place of saturated and *trans* fats in the diet.

THE MEDITERRANEAN DIET

The Mediterranean diet (one that is high in monounsaturated fat from olive oil and moderate in calories) made headlines when an Italian study appeared in the *Journal of the American Medical Association* in September 2004. The study followed two groups of 90 people who had metabolic syndrome (see "What Is Metabolic Syndrome?" on the next page) for two years. During the study, both groups increased their activity levels by 60 percent.

One study group was given detailed instructions about how to increase the whole grains, vegetables, fruits, nuts, and olive oil in their diets. The other 90 subjects consumed a "control" diet (50 percent to 60 percent of calories from carbohydrates, 15 percent to 20 percent of calories from protein, and less than 30 percent of calories from fat). After two years, those on the Mediterranean diet showed improvement in cholesterol levels, significantly less C-reactive protein in their blood, less insulin resistance, more weight loss, and improvements in the condition of their blood-vessel walls.

A follow-up study two years later revealed only 40 of the original 90 people on the Mediterranean diet still had metabolic syndrome, compared with 78 people in the control group.

WHAT IS METABOLIC SYNDROME?

Metabolic syndrome is a cluster of conditions that increases the risk of coronary artery disease and type 2 diabetes. In general, if a person has three or more of the conditions listed below, he or she likely has metabolic syndrome (which is sometimes called insulin-resistance syndrome).

- Excess weight, especially in the abdominal area
- High LDL cholesterol, low HDL cholesterol, and high triglyceride levels
- High blood pressure
- Insulin resistance (the body doesn't respond to insulin appropriately)
- "Thick" blood that is prone to clumping and clotting (as indicated by high levels of a substance called plasminogen activator inhibitor-1 in the blood)
- Inflamed blood vessels (as indicated by high levels in the blood of a compound named C-reactive protein)

MORE HEARTFELT EVIDENCE

A French study published in the *International Journal of Obesity-Related Metabolic Disorders* in June 2003 added to the evidence in favor of olive oil as a heart helper. Thirty-two people ate either a high-carbohydrate diet or one that was high in monounsaturated fat. After eight weeks, the people who consumed lots of monounsaturated fats had better triglyceride levels than those participants who were on the diet high in carbohydrates. Those who ate more monounsaturated fat also had less oxidative stress, a condition in which there are more free radicals than the body can handle and/or low levels of antioxidants. This condition puts the arteries at risk of damage and encourages heart disease (among other unhealthy effects).

The diet rich in monounsaturated fat also appeared to protect against smooth-muscle-cell proliferation, another risk factor for atherosclerosis.

Olive Oil—A Boon to Blood Pressure

An Italian study published in the December 2003 issue of the *Journal of Hypertension* reviewed numerous research projects that looked at various factors that affect blood pressure. The review indicated that unsaturated fat reduced blood pressure. The researchers went on to say that olive oil in particular was uniquely able to reduce high blood pressure—much more than sunflower oil.

A large study that appeared a year later in *The American Journal of Clinical Nutrition* looked at the diets of more than 20,000 Greeks who did not have high blood pressure when the study began. The study found that those who ate the typical Mediterranean diet had lower blood pressure. Further, when the effects of olive oil consumption were compared to those of vegetable oil consumption, olive oil was shown to have a more positive impact on blood pressure.

Spain is another country where olive oil is a staple in many households. People there typically use olive oil, sunflower oil (a mostly polyunsaturated oil), or a mixture of the two.

Researchers in one Spanish study wanted to learn the role each of these oils played in blood pressure, as well as how the oils held up to cultural cooking methods in which oil is heated to a high temperature for frying and later reused several times.

The study, which was published in the December 2003 issue of *The American Journal of Clinical Nutrition*, examined samples of cooking oil from the kitchens of 538 study participants. Researchers measured the blood pressure and conducted blood tests on those participants and nearly 500 more "control" subjects. Here's what they found:

- Olive oil was resistant to heat degradation.

- Mixed oil and sunflower oil degraded more than olive oil alone when heated and reused.

- Those who used sunflower oil, whether or not it had deteriorated, had higher blood pressure levels than those who used olive oil.

- The higher the monounsaturated fat consumption, the lower the blood pressure tended to be.

At the end of the study, the researchers concluded that because olive oil does a better job of maintaining its healthful properties and because it positively influences blood cholesterol and blood pressure levels, it should be the oil of choice in everyone's kitchen.

COOLING INFLAMMATION

Inflammation within the body may occur in response to cigarette smoking or eating large amounts of saturated fat and *trans* fat. In overweight or obese people, excess fat from fat cells can float through the bloodstream and cause inflammation. Although inflammation can help the body, it can also hurt.

Certain dietary fats cause more of an inflammatory response than others. *Trans* fat and the saturated fat in animal foods stimulate inflammation. To a smaller extent, polyunsaturated fat in foods such as safflower oil, sunflower oil, and corn oil trigger inflammation, as well. Again, this is where olive oil helps. Olive oil's phytonutrients—in this case phenolic compounds called squalene, beta-sitosterol, and tyrosol—don't cause the inflammation that other fats do.

WHAT IS INFLAMMATION?

Inflammation is the immune system's first line of defense against injury and infection. When an injury occurs, such as a simple cut on the finger, a set of events takes place within your body that forms a blood clot, fights infection, and begins the healing process. Inflammation is painful because blood vessels dilate upstream of the injury to bring more blood and nutrients to the injured area, but they constrict at the injury site. These actions result in fluids from the bloodstream pooling in tissue around the injury, which causes swelling and pressure that stimulate nerves and cause pain.

In some individuals, the immune system gets confused and begins to view some of the body's own healthy cells as "foreign invaders." It therefore directs an immune response—complete with inflammation—at healthy tissues, harming or even destroying them. This misdirected attack results in what's called an autoimmune disorder ("auto" meaning self). Rheumatoid arthritis and certain types of thyroid disease are autoimmune disorders. Asthma, too, is the result of inflammation gone awry.

When inflammation continues unabated for long periods of time, damage can occur in organs, such as the colon, or in blood vessels. Indeed, chronic inflammation within the body is looking more and more like a serious contributor to cardiovascular (heart and blood vessel) disease. Inflammation may damage the inner lining of blood vessels, which encourages plaque deposits to form. Inflammation may also cause plaque in arteries to break off and travel downstream, where it can become lodged and stop blood flow to a crucial artery that provides oxygen to important body parts, such as your heart or brain. When this happens, a heart attack or stroke (respectively) can occur.

Chronic inflammation within the body can wreak havoc on other body parts besides arteries. A team led by researchers at the Johns Hopkins Medical Institutions found that chronic inflammation of the colon might increase the risk of colon cancer. A ten-year study of more than 20,000 patients suggested a link between chronic inflammation and this disease, although a direct cause-and-effect relationship has not yet been established. These preliminary findings were discussed in the February 2004 edition of the *Journal of the American Medical Association*.

Scientists have discovered that inflammation can be reduced with low daily doses of aspirin or other nonsteroidal anti-inflammatory drugs (NSAIDs), which in turn appear to reduce the risk of diseases caused by inflammation. Fortunately, not only does olive oil not prompt the kind of inflammation other types of fat can, it actually has some ability to *reduce* inflammation, thanks to those helpful phytochemicals (squalene, beta-sitosterol, and tyrosol). So consuming olive oil on a regular basis may help decrease the risk of conditions linked to inflammation.

Yet another condition that appears to be linked to inflammation is type 2 diabetes, the most common form of diabetes that affects an estimated 20 million Americans. Having excess body fat seems to increase inflammation. As inflammation increases, so does insulin resistance. As insulin resistance increases, blood glucose levels rise and the risk of type 2 diabetes skyrockets.

What Is Oleocanthal and How Can It Help You?

An article published by Philadelphia researchers in the September 2005 issue of *Nature* identified a compound in olive oil called oleocanthal that has anti-inflammatory action. Their studies revealed that this compound can act like ibuprofen and other anti-inflammatory medications.

Olive oils differ widely in the amount of oleocanthal they possess. To get an idea of how oleocanthal-rich your olive oil of choice is, researchers suggest taking a sip of the oil to "see how strongly it stings the back of the throat." The stronger the sting, the more oleocanthal the oil contains. Fifty grams (nearly a quarter of a cup of olive oil) provides the same amount of anti-inflammatory action as 10 percent of the standard adult dose of ibuprofen.

Obviously, eating enough olive oil to equal a whole dose of ibuprofen is not a practical way to decrease your inflammation and pain. But consuming a moderate amount of olive oil daily—in place of most of the other fat you typically consume—over the long term may lessen chronic inflammation throughout the body and bloodstream. It might even somewhat diminish asthma and rheumatoid arthritis symptoms.

Future research will probably tell us more about olive oil's function in battling oxidation, inflammation, and all the multiple diseases and health conditions associated with them.

OLIVE OIL'S POSSIBLE ROLE IN CANCER PREVENTION

Many medical researchers believe cancers of the colon, prostate, and breast are linked to dietary fat intake. Typically, high-fat diets were blamed, but research is beginning to suggest the more important factor may be the type of fat in the diet. In Spain, Italy, and Greece, where olive oil is used in most households, cancer incidence is much lower than in northern Europe and the United States, where olive oil use isn't as widespread.

There is plenty of controversy regarding whether olive oil can play any part in helping to prevent breast cancer, but women who follow a Mediterranean-style diet appear to have a lower risk of the disease. A study published in the March 2005 issue of the *Annals of Oncology* showed that oleic acid, the principal monounsaturated fat in olive oil, dramatically decreased the growth of aggressive forms of breast tumors in test tubes. When oleic acid was combined with the commonly used breast cancer drug Herceptin, the effectiveness of the drug was vastly improved.

A review of studies conducted between 1990 and 2003 that was presented in the July 2005 issue of the *World Journal of Surgical Oncology* noted a direct association between saturated fat intake and breast cancer incidence. The more saturated fat consumed, the higher the incidence of breast cancer. In addition, the researchers reported an inverse relationship between the disease and oleic acid: The more oleic acid a woman ate, the lower her risk of breast cancer.

On the other hand, a different meta-analysis, published in the September 2004 *International Journal of Cancer*, analyzed ten studies that involved more than 2,000 cases of breast cancer. It found opposite results—the more oleic acid consumed, the higher the rate of breast cancer.

Clearly, more studies are needed to determine olive oil's real relationship to breast cancer. In the meantime, moderation may be the key to reaping the benefits of olive oil without increasing risk.

THE FRUIT'S LABOR

If you want to get olive oil's benefits from eating the fruit rather than the oil, just how many olives do you need to eat? There is about one tablespoon of oil in:

- ◆ 20 medium Mission olives
- ◆ 40 small black olives
- ◆ 20 jumbo black olives
- ◆ 7 colossal black olives

DIABETES AND OLIVE OIL

People living with diabetes have to work hard to keep their blood sugar, also called blood glucose, levels under control. One way to do so is to eat a diet that is fairly low in carbohydrates. Because people with diabetes are also at an elevated risk of developing heart disease, they are advised to limit their intake of dietary fat.

Lately, researchers and nutritionists have been debating the best type of eating pattern for people with diabetes. Some research indicates that a diet high in monounsaturated fat may be better than a low-fat, low-carbohydrate diet.

Numerous studies have suggested that people with diabetes who consume a diet high in monounsaturated fat have the same level of control over blood sugar levels as those who eat a low-fat diabetic diet. But monounsaturated fat also helps keep triglyceride levels in check, reduce LDL cholesterol levels, and increase HDL cholesterol levels.

Researchers in Spain published an article in *The American Journal of Clinical Nutrition* in September 2003 that concluded calorie-controlled diabetic diets high in monounsaturated fat do not cause weight gain and are more pleasing to eat than low-fat diets. The researchers determined that a diet high in monounsaturated fat is a good idea for people with diabetes.

Research is still inconsistent as to whether monounsaturated fat actually plays a role in stabilizing blood glucose levels, but evidence is leaning in that direction. A review of a number of studies, which was done by German researchers and appeared in the official journal of the German Diabetes Association, found that blood glucose levels were lower in people who ate a diet rich in monounsaturated fat than in people who ate a low-fat diet. Further, they said increasing monounsaturated-fat intake lowered LDL cholesterol levels in some, though not all, subjects.

WEIGHTY ISSUES

MARVELOUS POLYPHENOLS

Polyphenols are advantageous not only to human health but also to the health of the olive. Phenolic compounds protect the olive, prevent oxidation of its oil, and allow it to stay in good condition longer. In addition, they increase the shelf life of olive oil and contribute to its tart flavor.

Medical professionals are greatly concerned about the obesity problem in the United States. Obesity often comes hand-in-hand with high levels of cholesterol and lipids in the blood (hyperlipidemia), heart disease, high blood pressure, diabetes, certain cancers, and a higher rate of premature death.

Health-care professionals often recommend following a strict but healthy diet in order to lose weight. But there may be some good news for those overweight folks who struggle to limit dietary fat. Research suggests that replacing other types of fats with monounsaturated fat, especially olive oil, helps people lose a moderate amount of weight without additional food restriction or physical activity. So just imagine what adding a lower-calorie diet and increased physical activity (which is always a good idea) to the consumption of monounsaturated fats like olive oil could do for your weight-loss efforts.

FDA scientists reviewed many different studies when they evaluated whether to allow health claims for monounsaturated fat on food labels in 2003. The researchers wanted to ensure that a proposed recommendation to eat 13.5 grams (one table-spoon) of olive oil per day wouldn't contribute to weight gain in the American population. A number of studies showed that when people substituted monounsaturated-fat-rich olive oil for saturated fat, they either maintained their weight or lost weight. A diet high in monounsaturated fat and low in carbo-hydrates actually resulted in more weight loss than a low-fat, high-carbohydrate diet.

What's more, the FDA determined that eating 13.5 grams of monounsaturated fat in a dietary pattern low in saturated fat and cholesterol would reduce total blood cholesterol and LDL cholesterol levels by an average of 5 percent, resulting in a 10 percent decrease in coronary heart disease. However, the FDA did not approve this particular claim for food labels. Instead, the agency approved a stronger claim linking the consumption of 23 grams (about two tablespoons) of olive oil to a decreased risk of coronary heart disease. (See the "Now Read This!" sidebar on page 117 to read this claim.)

Another study showed that when people ate monounsaturated fat, they ate less. For example, when served bread with olive oil, participants ate 23 percent less bread than when they ate it with butter, a saturated fat. Scientists speculate that because monounsaturated fat is more satisfying than other types of fat, people eat less of it. Additionally, the body's metabolism of monounsaturated fat after a meal appears to be different from the metabolism of saturated fat. This difference in metabolism

DIET RIGHT

A study with exciting results appeared in the October 2005 issue of the *Archives of Internal Medicine.* In it, 65 people were divided into two groups and given two different diets for 12 weeks. One group received the diet recommended by the U.S. government's National Cholesterol Education Program, which replaces saturated fat with carbohydrates and is moderate in protein. The other group was given a "modified low-carbohydrate" (MLC) diet with the same amount of calories as the other diet, but lower in total carbohydrates and higher in protein, monounsaturated fat, and complex carbohydrates. (Complex carbohydrates are carbohydrates that contain fiber and are minimally processed, such as whole-grain foods, fruits, vegetables, and legumes.)

At the end of the study, those who received the diet rich in monounsaturated fat saw tremendous results:

◆ The MLC group lost significantly more weight (13.6 pounds vs. 7.5 pounds on average) than the other group.

◆ The MLC group saw significant, favorable changes in triglyceride levels and all types of cholesterol levels.

◆ The MLC group showed a reduction in waist-to-hip ratio (an indicator of amount of abdominal fat, which is linked to heart disease risk).

may be what causes slight weight loss. (Researchers haven't yet determined exactly how this works.)

Several other studies indicate that monounsaturated fat may even enhance the body's breakdown of stored fat. A study of rats that was published in the *British Journal of Nutrition* in December 2003 found that monounsaturated fat facilitated the release of fat from rats' fat cells. Also, insulin became less able to prevent the breakdown of fat, which made it easier for fat cells to release their stored fat for elimination by the body. Thus, an increase in monounsaturated fat in the diet (along with, presumably, an equivalent decrease in saturated-fat intake) may help with weight loss; results were opposite in the rats that were given polyunsaturated fat.

A pair of studies that were published in the *Asia-Pacific Journal of Clinical Nutrition* in 2004 looked at whether a diet high in monounsaturated fat was more effective for weight loss than a diet that was low in total fat. The studies also examined the effects of a Mediterranean diet on blood cholesterol and triglyceride levels.

The two studies tracked a total of 255 participants (155 in one study, 100 in the other) for 15 months. Researchers concluded that a Mediterranean diet was very effective for weight loss in the short term (3 months) *and* 15 months later. Participants who completed the study's initial three-month program had better weight-loss results and regained less weight after 15 months than those who did not complete the program. These results were comparable to or even better than the typical results found in studies of common weight-loss programs and combination diet/drug therapy.

NUTRIENT CONTENT OF OLIVE OIL

Nutrient	Amount in one tablespoon	Daily amount recommended for the average adult (if applicable)
Calories	119	2,000
Protein	0 g	46 g (women) 56 g (men)
Carbohydrates	0 g	130 g
Fiber	0 g	25 g (women) 38 g (men)
Total fat	13.5 g	65 g maximum
Monounsaturated fat	9.85 g	Not applicable
Polyunsaturated fat	1.421 g	Not applicable
Saturated fat	1.864 g	20 g
Cholesterol	0 g	300 mg
Phytosterol	30 g	2 g
Vitamin E	1.94 mg	2 g
Vitamin K	8.1 mcg	90 mcg (women) 120 mcg (men)
Iron	0.08 mg	18 mg (women) 8 mg (men)

g = grams, mg = milligrams, mcg = micrograms

Note: Olive oil is not a source of any vitamins other than vitamins E and K and is not a source of any mineral other than iron.

Source: U.S. Department of Agriculture, Agricultural Research Service. 2005. USDA National Nutrient Database for Standard Reference, Release 18. Nutrient Data Laboratory Home Page, www.ars.usda.gov/ba/bhnrc/ndl

The study also found that a Mediterranean diet had favorable effects on HDL cholesterol and triglyceride levels at three months and a neutral effect on total cholesterol and LDL cholesterol levels. (A neutral effect means there were no significant changes in these measurements.) In the study with 155 patients, HDL levels increased by 9.6 percent and triglyceride levels decreased by 31.6 percent.

In a small Australian study published in the *British Journal of Nutrition* in September 2003, eight men were given all their food and beverages for four weeks. Their meals and snacks were either high in saturated fat or high in monounsaturated fat. Later, the men switched diets. There were no significant differences in the amount of calories consumed or the amount of physical activity the men did. Yet the results showed that when the men substituted monounsaturated fat for saturated fat, they lost weight and body fat.

OH, THOSE POWERFUL OLIVES

Not all olives are created equal. Just as some varieties of apples are sweeter or more tart than others, different varieties of olives yield varying amounts of oil. Large black olives typically purchased in a can from the grocer's shelf may contain as little as 7 percent oil. These are table olives. At the other end of the spectrum, some olives contain up to 35 percent oil. These are the ones used for pressing.

No matter where the oil comes from, increasing the amount of olive oil in your diet is a great way to eat your way to good health. Find out how to replace your bad fats with olive oil in the next chapter.

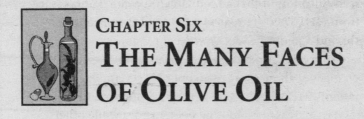

CHAPTER SIX
THE MANY FACES OF OLIVE OIL

A visit to the local market for olive oil may make your head spin. With dozens of choices, which one is best? Which has the most healing properties? Which is best right out of the bottle, and which is best for cooking? Fear not, because your olive oil IQ is about to increase.

Once you choose the olive oil that is right for you and your recipes, you must be careful using and storing it to preserve its healthful qualities. But you'll be rewarded for your careful selection and storage when you experience olive oil's aroma and flavor in your favorite dishes.

FROM TREE TO TABLE

The craft of turning olives into oil has been honed in the Mediterranean region over thousands of years, and techniques have been passed down from generation to generation. The process is truly a regional art. The method used in Greece is different from the one used in Spain, and each individual grower might have a unique way of tending the trees and producing the tasty liquid gold.

Mediterranean olive trees must mature for several years before they produce olives. Careful pruning optimizes the number of olives a single tree will bear. A meticulous hand is necessary because it takes at least ten pounds of olives to produce one liter (about four cups) of olive oil.

Hundreds of olive varieties exist, but only several dozen are grown commercially around the world. Some varieties are bursting with health-promoting polyphenols, while others contain few. The type of olive used to make any particular bottle of oil is rarely listed on the label. However, for those labels that do have the information, the following table, which shows which olives are richest in beneficial polyphenols, will be helpful.

Polyphenol Content of Selected Olive Varieties

VERY HIGH	HIGH	MEDIUM HIGH
Coratina	Bosana	Frantoio
Cornicabra	Chemlali	
Koroneiki	Manzanillo	
Moraiolo	Picholine	
Picual	Picholine marocaine	
	Verdial de huevar	

The time at which olives are harvested also plays a major role in flavor and polyphenol content. The peak time is a short period right as the olives ripen. Olives are at their prime for only about two or three weeks. Healthy compounds then rapidly diminish over the next two to five weeks.

PICKING PARTICULARS

It takes quite a bit of work to coax oil out of olives. Traditionally, trees were shaken or beaten with sticks to make the olives drop to the ground. Such tough treatment is not good for olives, however. Tumbling out of a tree and plopping onto the ground causes bruising. Soft fruits, such as peaches and plums, wouldn't take kindly to this type of treatment; they would bruise, too, and we would never think of harvesting them this way. Olives are also soft fruits that should be treated delicately because once they bruise, the beneficial oils within start to degrade.

Some olive oil labels declare that their bottles' contents are made from handpicked olives. This typically denotes a better-quality oil. Some growers separate their olives into "ground" olives (those collected from the ground) and "tree" olives (those picked from the tree) and use them for different grades of oil. Many large-scale growers use a tree-shaking device and set up nets beneath the trees that catch the olives before they hit the ground.

Growers must be careful when transporting olives from the trees to the processing plant. Olives are best carried in shallow containers so they don't pile up too deeply and crush one another. Any damage to the olives can trigger oxidation and fermentation, which create an "off" flavor. Olives should be processed soon after harvest because storing them also diminishes their quality.

PRESS TIME

After olives are picked, any leaves, twigs, and stems are removed, and the olives are washed. Then it's time for pressing. Back in the old days, processors used stone or granite wheels to crush the olives. Today, stainless steel rollers crush the olives and pits and grind them into paste. The paste then undergoes malaxation, a process in which water is slowly stirred into the paste. Malaxation allows the tiny oil molecules to clump together and concentrate.

The mixture is stirred for 20 to 40 minutes. Longer mixing times increase oil production and give the oil a chance to pick up additional flavors from the olive paste. However, the mixing also exposes the oil to air, producing free radicals that poorly affect its quality.

Modern systems use closed mixing chambers filled with a harmless gas to prevent oxidation. This method increases yield and flavor and preserves quality. The mixture may be heated to about 82 degrees

PRIZED FRUIT

Olives and olive oil were so valued in ancient Greece that they were given as awards to Olympic athletes. A wreath of olive leaves was placed on the heads of winning athletes, and their prize might be an amphora (a two-handled jug with a narrow neck) filled with olive oil.

LABEL LINGO

Here are some terms you might see on olive oil labels that describe extraction methods. The first two are cold-extraction processes. Olive oils processed by these methods retain the vitamins, health-boosting phytochemicals, color, flavor, and aroma of the olives. The second two are heat-extraction processes. The heat used in these techniques takes a toll on olive oil. Excessive heat destroys many of the fragile nutrients and phytochemicals and just about all of the color, flavor, and aroma.

Cold pressed. This method removes the oil from olives through pressing and grinding. For the oil to be labeled "cold pressed," the heat generated by friction from the grinding must not exceed 86 degrees Fahrenheit. (Other oils, such as safflower and canola, are sometimes cold pressed, but for those oils, friction temperatures of up to 120 degrees Fahrenheit are allowed.)

Vacuum extraction. This is a cold-extraction method done in the absence of air and light at temperatures as low as 70 degrees Fahrenheit. Olives are crushed and ground, then mixed with water and churned in a device that uses a vacuum. The process ensures no air is introduced into the system and preserves the antioxidants and nutrients.

Expeller pressed. This method also uses grinding and pressing, but with extreme amounts of pressure, sometimes up to 15 tons per square inch. This intense amount of pressure creates a lot of heat and friction that takes the oil to temperatures of up to 300 degrees Fahrenheit.

Solvent extraction. This technique uses chemicals, such as hexane, to remove oil from olives. The oil is then boiled to get rid of the chemicals. The oil may then undergo additional heat processing, bleaching, or deodorizing, which leads to a bland oil, but one with a high smoke point and long shelf life.

Fahrenheit, which further increases yield but does allow some oxidation. This temperature is low enough to be considered "cold pressed."

Next, the paste is put on mats and further pressed or sent through a centrifuge (a compartment that is rotated on a central axis at extreme speed to separate materials). When the centrifuge spins, the olive paste remnants are pushed to the sides of the compartment cylinder while water and oil are extracted from the center of the centrifuge. The oil and water are later separated.

The solid material that remains after the extraction of the oil is called pomace, and it contains residual oil. Some manufacturers will use steam, hexane, or other solvents to squeeze more oil out of the pomace. This low-quality oil must be labeled as pomace oil.

Oil may then be refined, bleached, and/or deodorized. Refining reduces acidity and any bitter taste. Bleaching removes chlorophyll and carotenoids (naturally occurring pigments that give plants their colors) and possibly pesticides, resulting in a light-colored oil with fewer nutrients. Deodorizing removes the fragrant aroma of the olive oil.

In the manufacturing plant, oil is stored in stainless steel containers at about 65 degrees Fahrenheit to prevent breakdown before it is bottled and shipped.

OLIVE OIL OPTIONS

Rich, beautiful, and fragrant, olive oil is much like wine—taste is a matter of personal preference. The many variables that go into the production of olive oil yield dramatic differences in color, aroma, and flavor. The following factors impact the taste of olive oil:

- Variety of olive used
- Location and soil conditions where the olives were grown
- Environmental factors and weather during the growing season
- Olive ripeness
- Timing of the harvest
- Harvesting method
- Length of time between the harvest and pressing
- Pressing technique
- Packaging and storage methods

Olive oils are graded by production method, acidity content, and flavor. The International Olive Oil Council (IOOC) sets

FREE ACIDS ARE BAD ACIDS

An olive oil's quality is determined by the amount of acidity, or free oleic acid, in the oil. Higher-quality oils have lower acidity levels.

Wait, didn't we say in the last chapter that oleic acid has beneficial health properties? Yes, it does, but it is *free* oleic acid (a type of fatty acid) that indicates lesser quality. Oleic acid can either roam around by itself as a single fatty acid or it can be attached to other fat components.

To understand what this means, picture a capital letter "E." The vertical line of the "E" is the backbone—a triglyceride, that common type of fat. Each of the three horizontal arms of the "E" contains a fatty acid, one or more of them being oleic acid. In this form, attached to the triglyceride, oleic acid is valuable. But if the oleic acid arm of the "E" triglyceride breaks off, it becomes free, or unbound, and is therefore called "free oleic acid."

Difficult growing conditions; olives picked too soon or too late; infestations of pests, such as olive flies; fungal diseases; damage or bruising during harvesting; and poor storage conditions all allow free oleic acid to form. When this happens, the oil begins to break down, diminishing its quality.

quality standards that most olive-oil-producing countries use, but the United States does not legally recognize these benchmarks. Instead, the U.S. Department of Agriculture uses a different system that was set up before the IOOC existed. However, American olive growers and oil importers are encouraging the USDA to adopt standards similar to those of the IOOC.

WHERE IN THE WORLD?

When buying olive oil, you'll see varieties from all over the globe. Most of the world's supply is produced from olives grown in Spain, Italy, and Greece, but other areas, including France and California, are in on the fun, too. Here's what you need to know about olive oil and geography:

◆ Spanish olive oil is typically golden yellow with a fruity, nutty flavor. Spain produces about 45 percent of the world's olive supply.

◆ Italian olive oil is often dark green and has an herbal aroma and a grassy flavor. Italy grows about 20 percent of the world's olives.

◆ Greek olive oil packs a strong flavor and aroma and tends to be green. Greece produces about 13 percent of the world's olive supply.

◆ French olive oil is typically pale in color and has a milder flavor than other varieties.

◆ Californian olive oil is light in color and flavor, with a bit of a fruity taste.

Olives from different countries are often blended together to produce an oil variety. Or, olives from diverse areas of one country may be combined. These bulk-blended oils are the most economical but are still high quality. On the other hand, some producers only use olives that are grown in a specific area of a country. These regional oils are usually known for their unique flavors.

Estate olive oils are the cream of the crop. Estate oils are produced using olives from a single olive farm. These olives are usually handpicked, then pressed and bottled right at the estate. Expect to get the best flavor out of these varieties, but also expect to pay more.

MAKING THE GRADES

There are three basic grades of edible olive oil, and several types within each grade. Extra virgin includes "premium extra virgin" and "extra virgin"; virgin comprises "fine virgin," "virgin," and "semifine virgin"; and olive oil includes what used to be called "pure olive oil" and "refined oil."

All types of extra-virgin and virgin oils are made from the first pressing of the olives, which removes about 90 percent of the olives' juice. Chemicals and high heat are not allowed in the production of extra-virgin or virgin oils—no further processing or refining occurs after the pressing process. Neither extra-virgin nor virgin oils are allowed to contain any refined olive oil.

Virgin olive oils. At the head of the olive oil class sit the extra-virgins, followed closely by the virgins. The difference between two oils and where they rank in the following hierarchy may be just half a percentage point of acidity. However, that is all it takes to distinguish between a very good oil and a great oil.

NATURE'S PERFECT COMBINATION

Although the amount and type of oil in olives depends on their variety and growing conditions, in general, the olive offers a perfect ratio of the healthy fats.

- Oleic acid is a monounsaturated fat and is the predominant type of oil in olive oil. Oleic acid accounts for 55 percent to 85 percent of an olive oil's content.

- Linoleic acid is an omega-6 polyunsaturated fat. It makes up about 9 percent to 10 percent of a typical olive oil.

- Linolenic acid is a heart-healthy omega-3 polyunsaturated fat. The average olive oil is about 1 percent linolenic acid.

- Saturated fat and other substances, such as vitamins, phytochemicals, moisture, and other trace compounds comprise the rest of the oil in an olive.

As discussed in chapter five, you can see that olives offer the government's recommended omega-6-to-omega-3 ratio of 10-to-1.

"Premium extra-virgin olive oil" is nature's finest, thanks to its extremely low acidity (possibly as low as 0.225 percent). It is best suited for using uncooked in dishes where you can appreciate its exquisite aroma and flavor. Try it in salads, as a dip for bread, or as a condiment.

"Extra-virgin olive oil" has a fruity taste and may be pale yellow to bright green in color. In general, the deeper the color, the more flavor it yields. IOOC regulations say extra-virgin olive oil must have a superior flavor and contain no more than 0.8 percent acidity, but other regulators set the acidity cut-off point at 1 percent. As with the premium version, it is best to use extra-virgin olive oil uncooked in order to appreciate its flavor.

"Fine virgin olive oil" must have a "good" taste (as judged by IOOC standards) and an acidity level of no more than 1.5 percent. Fine virgin olive oil is less expensive than extra-virgin oil but is close in quality and is good uncooked.

SHOPPING FOR OIL

High-quality oils are available in some grocery stores, specialty shops, and mail-order catalogs as well as on the Internet. Be prepared to spend anywhere from $10 to $40 for a half-liter (a little more than two cups) of high-quality oil. Some shops and distributors offer an "olive oil of the month" club in which they ship you a specialty olive oil monthly.

"Virgin olive oil" must have a "good" taste, and its acidity must be 2 percent or less. Like other virgin oils, it cannot contain any refined oil. Virgin olive oil is good for cooking, but it also has enough flavor to be enjoyed uncooked.

"Semifine virgin olive oil" must have an acidity no higher than 3.3 percent. It is good for cooking but doesn't have enough flavor to be enjoyed uncooked.

Lower-quality oils. Some olive oil is further refined after the first pressing. These three types of oils can no longer bear the title "virgin."

When virgin oils are not fit for human consumption (because of poor flavor, an acidity level greater than 3.3 percent, or an unpleasant aroma), they are sent to a processing plant where they become "refined olive oils." There they undergo processing with agents that might include heat, chemicals, and/or filtration. These refined olive oils become clear, odorless, and flavorless and have an acidity level of 0.3 percent or less, which gives them a long shelf life (refined olive oils' only real advantage). They are typically blended with virgin oils, used in cooking, or used for foods that are labeled "packed in olive oil."

The current "olive oil" category used to be called "pure olive oil." Today, oils in this classification are a blend of refined olive oil and a virgin olive oil. The virgin oil lends a little aroma and flavor to the final product, which can have an acidity level of no more than 1.5 percent. In most cases, oils in this category contain about 85 percent refined oil and 15 percent virgin or extra-virgin oil. Oils of the "olive oil" grade withstand heat well.

"Olive pomace oil" is made from the olive paste that is left in the centrifuge after the olives are pressed and the oil-water mixture is extracted. Olive pomace oil can be treated with heat and chemicals to extract additional oil (about 10 percent of the original amount of oil in the olives). Its acidity cannot exceed 1.5 percent. Virgin oil may be added to pomace oil for color and flavor. Olive pomace oil is edible, but it may not carry the

ORGANIC OLIVE OIL

All plants have natural enemies, and olive trees are no different. Olives are susceptible to a pest known as the olive fly, which lives inside the olive and makes a feast of the fruit. Fungus is another adversary of olives, although olive flies are a bigger threat. Growers use pesticides, fungicides, and herbicides to protect their crops when necessary. If you'd like to avoid these chemicals, buy organic olive oil.

In the United States there are strict guidelines governing the use of the term "organic" on labels. If the label says "USDA Certified Organic," the producer has proven to the U.S. Department of Agriculture that the oil is made with olives that were grown without chemicals, among other requirements. The regulations apply whether the olives are grown and bottled in the United States or imported from other countries.

name "olive oil." This oil is most often used commercially and is rarely seen on the grocer's shelf.

Other oils. Sometimes, cooks don't need the full flavor of olive oil, or they need a little extra taste added. Oil producers have responded to these needs by creating lite olive oil and flavored oils.

"Lite olive oil" is also called "light" or "mild" oil. These oils have undergone an extremely fine filtration process (without the use of heat or chemicals) to remove most of the natural color, aroma, and flavor. This makes them suitable for cooking or baking in recipes in which a fruity olive flavor isn't needed. The terms "lite," "light," and "mild" can be used along with "extra virgin olive oil," "virgin olive oil," and "olive oil."

In this case, "lite" or "light" do not refer to fat content. These oils contain the same amount of fat and calories as any other olive oil (about 13 grams of fat and 120 calories per table-spoon). The classifications instead refer to the oil's lighter color and flavor.

Do you want oil with more flavor rather than less? Some manu-facturers make high-quality flavored olive oils by adding sweet or savory ingredients, such as spices, herbs, vegetables, or citrus peel, to extra-virgin oils during the pressing process. Lower-quality flavored oils have these ingredients added after pressing.

Commercially prepared flavored oils are usually safe to keep and use for a long period of time, but homemade ones are not. If you create your own homemade flavored oils, make only small amounts that you can use within several days, and always store them in the refrigerator to prevent the growth of poten-tially harmful bacteria. The oil itself does not support bacterial growth, but the moisture and nutrients in fresh herbs, garlic, dried tomatoes, or citrus peels do.

COLOR CONSIDERATIONS

Green olive oils come from unripe olives and impart a slightly bitter, pungent flavor. Emerald-tinged oils have fruity, grassy, and peppery flavors that dominate the foods in which you use

Are you wishing for a vacation to a warm, distant land but you can't get away? Open a bottle of quality olive oil and your senses will think you're there. When you smell olive oil's fruity, heady aroma and get a taste of the exquisite flavor, you can almost see the majestic olive trees growing on a hillside beneath the Tuscan sun.

them. These oils are great with neutral-flavored foods that allow their bold flavors to shine. You can pair green olive oils with strongly flavored foods as long as they complement the oils' pungent tastes.

Olive oils that glimmer with a golden color are made from ripe olives. Olives turn from green to bluish-purple to black as they ripen. Oils made from ripe olives have a milder, smoother, somewhat buttery taste without bitterness. These oils are perfect for foods with subtle flavors because the gentle taste of a ripe olive oil won't overshadow mildly flavored foods.

STORAGE

Because of olive oil's high monounsaturated fat content, it can be stored longer than most other oils—as long as it's stored properly. Oils are fragile and need to be treated gently to preserve their healthful properties and to keep them from becoming a health hazard full of free radicals.

When choosing your storage location, remember that heat, air, and light are the enemies of oil. These elements help create free radicals, which eventually lead to excessive oxidation and

MORE THAN BAD TASTE

Rancid oils may not please the palate, but they're really bad news for your body. They damage cell membranes; may decrease immune function; and are linked to heart disease, cancer, and other degenerative diseases. What's more, rancidity diminishes nutrient quality.

Heat, air, and light cause oxidation in olive oil, but so do the oil's aging process and enzymes that are naturally present. Many of the nutrients in olive oils are antioxidants, such as vitamin E, but as the oil ages or experiences other oxidative stress, these antioxidants break down. The oil deteriorates very rapidly when most of the antioxidants are gone. If bottles of oil in your kitchen have been sitting in the light at room temperature for more than a couple of months, discard them.

rancidity in the oil that will leave a bad taste in your mouth. Even worse, oxidation and free radicals contribute to heart disease and cancer.

Rancidity can set in long before you can taste it or smell it. Rotten oils harm cells and use up precious antioxidants. Even though rancid oil doesn't pose a food-safety type of health risk, the less you consume, the better.

The best storage containers for olive oil are made of either tinted glass (to keep out light) or a nonreactive metal, such as stainless steel. Avoid metal containers made of iron or copper because the chemical reactions between the olive oil and those metals create toxic compounds. Avoid most plastic, too; oil can absorb noxious substances such as polyvinyl chlorides (PVCs) out of the plastic. Containers also need a tight cap or lid to keep out unwanted air.

KEEP IT COOL

Temperature is also important in preventing degradation of olive oil. Experts recommend storing the oil at 57 degrees Fahrenheit, the temperature of a wine cellar. Aren't lucky

BRIGHT LIGHTS, BIG PROBLEMS

Light destroys oils, and unfortunately, many olive oils are sold in clear glass containers. Most grocery stores have bright lights that beat down on shelves throughout the day, and oils sold in stores that are open 24 hours never get a reprieve from the light. In a busy store, oils sell quickly and are not subjected to all that light for very long, but that might not be the case in stores that don't get much traffic or don't rotate their stock very often.

Avoid choosing bottles covered in dust (that's a sure sign they've been on the shelf for quite a while). Bottles on the top shelf or in the front of a display are also subjected to more of the damaging rays. When shopping, grab a bottle from the back of the display, where direct light doesn't reach. Some olive oil producers use green or brown bottles to keep out the light; these are the wisest choice.

enough to have a wine cellar? A room temperature of about 70 degrees Fahrenheit will be fine. If your kitchen is routinely warmer than that, you can refrigerate the oil.

In fact, refrigeration is best for long-term storage of all olive oils except premium extra-virgin ones. Consider keeping small amounts of olive oil in a sealed container at room temperature—perhaps in a small, capped porcelain jug that keeps out air and light. This way, your olive oil is instantly ready to use. Keep the rest in the refrigerator, but remember that refrigerated olive oil will solidify and turn cloudy, making it difficult to use. Returning it to room temperature restores its fluidity and color.

FREEZING OLIVE OIL

If you need to store your oil for a long period of time, stick it in the freezer. Believe it or not, olive oil freezes well, retaining its health properties and flavor. However, its complex mixture of oils and waxes prevent it from freezing at exactly 32 degrees Fahrenheit. Folk wisdom says you can tell the quality of an olive oil from the temperature at which it freezes, but this is not true.

Another option is to store olive oil in a wide-mouth glass jar in the refrigerator. Even though it solidifies, you can easily spoon out any amount you need. A clear jar is fine because it's dark inside the refrigerator most of the time.

If you don't want to refrigerate your olive oil, keep it in a dark, cool cupboard away from the stove or other heat-producing appliances. Olive oil connoisseurs recommend storing premium extra-virgin olive oils at room temperature. If refrigerated, condensation could develop and adversely affect their flavor. Refrigeration does not affect the quality or flavor of other olive oils.

Olive oil will keep well if stored in a sealed container in a cool, dark cupboard for about one year. If unopened, the oil may keep for as long as two years.

Older Isn't Better

Unlike wine, oil does not improve with age. As olive oil gets older, it gradually breaks down, more free oleic acid is formed, the acidity level rises, and flavor weakens. Extra-virgin oils keep better because they have a low acidity level to start with, but you should use lower-quality oils within months because they start out with higher acidity levels. As oil sits on your shelf, its acidity level rises daily, and soon it is not palatable.

You'll get the best quality and flavor from your olive oil if you use it within a year of pressing. Olive oil remains at its peak for about two or three months after pressing, but unfortunately, few labels carry bottling dates or "use by" dates, let alone pressing dates.

More is at issue than flavor, however. Research shows the nutrients in olive oil degrade over time. In a study that appeared in the May 2004 issue of the *Journal of Agriculture and Food Chemistry*, Spanish researchers tested virgin olive oil that had been stored for 12 months under perfect conditions. What they found was quite surprising: After 12 months, many of the oil's prime healing substances had practically vanished. All the vitamin E was gone, as much as 30 percent of the chlorophyll had deteriorated, and 40 percent of the beta-

carotene had disintegrated.
Phenol levels had dropped
dramatically, too.

THE STORAGE BOTTOM LINE

The morals of the story when it comes to olive oil storage are:

◆ If possible, determine the age of the olive oil you're buying, or buy from a store where product turnover is rapid.

◆ Store your olive oil in an airtight container in a dark place at room temperature. You can refrigerate or freeze most oils for long-term storage.

◆ Buy small amounts that you can use within a few months.

OLIVE OIL IN THE KITCHEN

Olive oil helps carry the flavor of foods and spices, provides a pleasing feel in the mouth, and satisfies the appetite. Liberal use of it will enhance both savory and sweet dishes without guilt because of its wonderful health-boosting properties (although if you're trying to lose weight, you may not want to overdo it, because like all fats, it provides nine calories per gram). Virgin and extra-virgin oils are best used uncooked or cooked at low to medium temperatures. Refined and olive oil grade oils are the choices for high-heat uses, such as frying.

An oil's smoke point is the temperature at which it smokes when heated. Any oil is ruined at its smoke point and is no longer good for you. If you heat an oil to its smoke point, carefully discard it and start over. Olive oil has a higher smoke point than most other oils (about 400 degrees Fahrenheit). Refined olive oils have a slightly higher smoke point (about 410 degrees Fahrenheit).

Tips for Cooking with Olive Oil

Although extra-virgin and virgin olive oils stand up to heat remarkably well, they do lose flavor as they're heated, so they are best for uncooked dishes. Use them to harmonize the spices in a dish, to enhance and build flavors, and to add body and depth. Olive oil also balances the acidity in high-acid foods, such as tomatoes, vinegar, wine, and lemon juice. In general, treat your olive oils as you do your wines, carefully pairing their tastes with the flavors of the other ingredients in the dishes you are creating.

Here are some ways to use olive oil:

- Drizzle it over salad or mix it into salad dressing.
- Use in marinades or sauces for meat, fish, poultry, and vegetables. Oil penetrates nicely into the first few layers of the food being marinated.
- Add at the end of cooking for a burst of flavor.
- Drizzle over cooked pasta or vegetables.
- Use instead of butter or margarine as a healthy dip for bread. Pour a little olive oil into a small side dish and add a few splashes of balsamic vinegar, which will pool in the middle and look very attractive.
- For an easy appetizer, toast baguette slices under the broiler, rub them lightly with a cut clove of garlic, and add a little drizzle of olive oil.

- Replace butter with olive oil in mashed potatoes or on baked potatoes. For the ultimate mashed potatoes, whip together cooked potatoes, roasted garlic, and olive oil; season to taste.

- Make a tasty, heart-healthy dip by mixing cooked white beans, garlic, and olive oil in a food processor; season to taste with your favorite herbs.

- Use olive oil in your sauces—whisking will help emulsify, or blend, the watery ingredients with the oil in the sauce.

THE MOST VERSATILE VERSION

You can use multipurpose fine virgin olive oil in almost any recipe. It is moderately priced despite being close in flavor to more expensive extra-virgin olive oils. Plus, you can use it in high-heat applications, so feel free to grab fine virgin olive oil when you need to sauté, panfry, or stir-fry. Fine virgin olive oil is also the right choice when you want quality flavor but not that strong olive taste. Try these tips for fine virgin olive oil in your kitchen:

- Brush it on meats before grilling or broiling to seal in the meat flavor and juices and create a crispy exterior.

- Add to eggs and drizzle over toast.

- Sprinkle on brown rice.

- Before refrigerating homemade pesto, add a thin layer of fine virgin olive oil on top of the sauce after putting it in a jar so the pesto will keep its green color.

BAKING WITH OLIVE OIL

Most people don't think of using olive oil when baking, but it's actually a great way to get more monounsaturated fat and polyphenolic compounds in your diet. Choose the lite, light, or mild type of olive oil for baking, especially savory breads and

TURNING UP THE HEAT?

Whether you're sautéing, stir-frying, panfrying, or deep-frying, use olive oil and this advice to make your high-heat cooking great:

◆ Always heat the skillet or pan on medium-high heat before adding oil.

◆ When the skillet is hot, add olive oil and let it heat up to just below the smoke point before adding your food. This should take 30 to 90 seconds, depending on the heat of the burner and quality of the pan. When you place food in the pan, it should sizzle; if not, the pan and oil are not hot enough.

◆ Always pat food dry before putting it into hot oil; otherwise, a layer of steam will form between the food and the oil, making it difficult to get a good, scared, crispy exterior.

◆ When grilling or broiling, brush meats or vegetables with olive oil to enhance flavor, seal in juices, and make the outer surface crispy.

◆ Use the lower-quality olive-oil-grade stuff for panfrying, stir-frying, and deep-frying. Although it doesn't have much flavor, it does hold its heat well.

Simple Decadence

This recipe may sound odd, but it's delicious. Slice a baguette in quarter-inch slices, then top each with a square of high-quality bittersweet chocolate. Drizzle with lite extra-virgin olive oil and sprinkle with a bit of coarse sea salt. Bake at 350 degrees Fahrenheit for three to five minutes until the chocolate is melted. Add a little more olive oil and salt. Serve and melt your troubles away.

sweets such as cakes, cookies, and other desserts. Because of the filtration these types of oils have undergone, they withstand high-heat cooking methods.

Substituting olive oil for butter dramatically reduces the amount of fat—especially saturated fat—in your baked goods. And of course, olive oil does not contain any of butter's cholesterol. You'll also use less fat—you can substitute three tablespoons of olive oil for a quarter-cup of butter. (Check your cookbook for substituting advice.) The product still turns out as expected, but with 25 percent less fat, fewer calories, and more heart-healthy nutrients.

Healthy Combinations

The world is fortunate that nature provides such scrumptious foods abundant in healing properties. Olive oil, garlic, and vinegar complement each other in flavor and health benefits. Together, they make for culinary delights and healthy bodies. Enjoy them in good health!

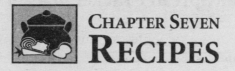

CHAPTER SEVEN
RECIPES

Enjoy this fabulous selection of great-tasting recipes featuring garlic, olive oil and vinegar.

Bruschetta

1 teaspoon olive oil
1 cup thinly sliced onion
½ cup chopped seeded tomato
2 tablespoons capers
¼ teaspoon black pepper
3 cloves garlic, finely chopped
1 teaspoon olive oil
4 slices French bread
½ cup (2 ounces) shredded reduced-fat Monterey Jack cheese

1. Heat oil in large nonstick skillet over medium heat until hot. Add onion; cook and stir 5 minutes. Stir in tomato, capers and pepper. Cook 3 minutes.

2. Preheat broiler. Combine garlic and olive oil in small bowl. Brush bread slices with mixture. Top with onion mixture; sprinkle with cheese. Place on baking sheet. Broil 3 minutes or until cheese melts.   *Makes 4 appetizer servings*

Nutrients per Serving: Calories: 90 (20% of calories from fat), Total Fat: 2 g, Saturated Fat: <1 g, Cholesterol: 0 mg, Sodium: 194 mg, Carbohydrate: 17 g, Dietary Fiber: <1 g, Protein: 3 g
Dietary Exchanges: 1 Starch, ½ Lean Meat

Bean Spread Cracker Stackers

1 can (15 ounces) kidney beans, rinsed and drained
1 tablespoon cider vinegar
1 tablespoon sour cream
2 teaspoons dried parsley
2 teaspoons (or 2 cloves) crushed garlic
½ teaspoon salt
½ teaspoon ground cumin
½ teaspoon hot pepper sauce
90 baked whole-wheat snack crackers

1. Place beans, vinegar, sour cream, parsley, garlic, salt, cumin and hot sauce in food processor or blender; process until smooth. Transfer bean mixture to bowl; cover and refrigerate at least 1 hour to allow flavors to blend.

2. To make stackers, spread 1 cracker with 1 teaspoon bean dip; top with second cracker, spreading the cracker with 1 teaspoon bean dip. Top with third cracker. Repeat with remaining bean mixture and crackers. Serve immediately.

Makes 15 appetizer servings

Tip: If you don't want to make all of the stackers at once, refrigerate the bean spread and keep on hand for up to one week. You can also use the bean spread as a dip with baked tortilla chips.

Nutrients per Serving (2 stackers): Calories: 134 (27% of calories from fat), Total Fat: 4 g, Saturated Fat: 2 g, Cholesterol: 0 mg, Sodium: 270 mg, Carbohydrate: 22 g, Dietary Fiber: 4 g, Protein: 4 g
Dietary Exchanges: 2 Starch

Fresh Tomato Eggplant Spread

1 medium eggplant
2 large ripe tomatoes, seeded and chopped
1 cup minced zucchini
¼ cup chopped green onions
2 tablespoons red wine vinegar
1 tablespoon finely chopped fresh basil
1 tablespoon olive oil
2 teaspoons finely chopped fresh oregano
1 teaspoon finely chopped fresh thyme
1 teaspoon honey
1 clove garlic, minced
⅛ teaspoon black pepper
¼ cup pine nuts or slivered almonds
32 melba toast rounds

1. Preheat oven to 375°F. Poke holes in eggplant with fork. Place in shallow baking pan. Bake 20 to 25 minutes or until tender. Cool completely. Peel and discard skin; finely chop eggplant. Place in colander; press to squeeze out excess liquid.

2. Combine eggplant, tomatoes, zucchini, green onions, vinegar, basil, oil, oregano, thyme, honey, garlic and pepper in large bowl. Mix well. Refrigerate 2 hours to allow flavors to blend.

3. Stir in pine nuts just before serving. Serve with melba toast rounds.   *Makes 8 appetizer servings*

Nutrients per Serving: Calories: 117 (31% of calories from fat), Total Fat: 4 g, Saturated Fat: 0 g, Cholesterol: 0 mg, Sodium: 65 mg, Carbohydrate: 15 g, Dietary Fiber: 2 g, Protein: 4 g
Dietary Exchanges: 1 Starch, 3 Vegetable

Red Pepper & Cheddar Crostini

1 (1-pound) narrow loaf French bread
3 tablespoons olive oil
1 teaspoon minced garlic
1 cup roasted red peppers (blotted dry if canned)
¼ cup (lightly packed) grated CABOT® Extra Sharp
    Cheddar
1 tablespoon capers, well drained
    Salt and ground black pepper to taste
2 hard-boiled eggs, finely chopped
2 tablespoons finely chopped fresh parsley

1. Preheat broiler. Cut bread into thin slices and arrange in single layer on baking sheets.

2. In small bowl, combine olive oil and garlic; brush mixture on tops of bread slices. Broil one sheet at a time until golden.

3. In food processor or blender, combine red peppers, cheese and capers; pulse until chopped but not pureed. Season with salt and pepper. In small bowl, combine chopped eggs and parsley.

4. Place heaping teaspoon of topping on each crostini and sprinkle with some of chopped egg mixture.

Makes about 32 crostini

Nutrients per Serving (1 crostini): Calories: 122 (36% of calories from fat), Total Fat: 5 g, Saturated Fat: 1 g, Cholesterol: 29 mg, Sodium: 355 mg, Carbohydrate: 15 g, Dietary Fiber: <1 g, Protein: 4 g
Dietary Exchanges: 1 Starch, 1 Fat

Roasted Garlic
Spread with Three Cheeses

2 medium heads garlic
2 packages (8 ounces each) fat-free cream cheese, softened
1 package (3½ ounces) goat cheese
2 tablespoons (1 ounce) crumbled blue cheese
1 teaspoon dried thyme
    Assorted sliced fresh vegetables
    Fresh thyme and red bell pepper (optional)

1. Preheat oven to 400°F. Cut tops off garlic heads to expose tops of cloves. Place garlic in small baking pan; bake 45 minutes or until very tender. Remove from pan; cool completely. Squeeze garlic into small bowl, discarding skins; mash garlic with fork.

2. Beat cream cheese and goat cheese in small bowl until smooth; stir in blue cheese, garlic and thyme. Cover; refrigerate 3 hours or overnight.

3. Spoon dip into serving bowl; serve with cucumbers, radishes, carrots and yellow bell peppers. Garnish with fresh thyme and red bell pepper, if desired.

Makes 21 appetizer servings

Nutrients per Serving (2 tablespoons spread): Calories: 37 (29% of calories from fat), Total Fat: 1 g, Saturated Fat: <1 g, Cholesterol: 9 mg, Sodium: 157 mg, Carbohydrate: 2 g, Dietary Fiber: <1 g, Protein: 4 g
Dietary Exchanges: ½ Lean Meat

Balsamic Chicken

1½ teaspoons fresh rosemary, minced *or* ½ teaspoon dried
   rosemary
  2 cloves garlic, minced
  ¾ teaspoon black pepper
  ½ teaspoon salt
  6 boneless skinless chicken breast halves
  1 tablespoon olive oil
  ¼ cup balsamic vinegar

1. Combine rosemary, garlic, pepper and salt in small bowl; mix well. Place chicken in large bowl; drizzle chicken with oil and rub with spice mixture. Cover and refrigerate several hours.

2. Preheat oven to 450°F. Spray heavy roasting pan or cast iron skillet with nonstick cooking spray. Place chicken in pan; bake 10 minutes. Turn chicken over, stirring in 3 to 4 tablespoons water if drippings begin to stick to pan.

3. Bake about 10 minutes or until chicken is golden brown and no longer pink in center. If pan is dry, stir in another 1 to 2 tablespoons water to loosen drippings.

4. Drizzle vinegar over chicken in pan. Transfer chicken to plates. Stir liquid in pan; drizzle over chicken. Garnish, if desired. *Makes 6 entrée servings*

Nutrients per Serving: Calories: 174 (29% of calories from fat), Total Fat: 5 g, Saturated Fat: 1 g, Cholesterol: 73 mg, Sodium: 242 mg, Carbohydrate: 3 g, Dietary Fiber: 1 g, Protein: 27 g
Dietary Exchanges: 3 Lean Meat

Beef Kabobs with Zucchini and Cherry Tomatoes

Marinade
- ¼ cup FILIPPO BERIO® Olive Oil
- 2 tablespoons chopped fresh parsley
- 2 tablespoons red wine vinegar
- 1 clove garlic, minced
- ½ teaspoon salt
- ⅛ teaspoon freshly ground black pepper

Kabobs
- 1 pound lean beef top sirloin or top round steak, well trimmed and cut into 1-inch cubes
- 1 small zucchini, cut into ½-inch-thick slices
- 12 cherry tomatoes
- 6 metal skewers

In medium glass bowl or dish, whisk together olive oil, parsley, vinegar, garlic, salt and pepper. Add steak, zucchini and tomatoes; toss until lightly coated. Cover; marinate in refrigerator 2 hours or overnight. Drain meat and vegetables, reserving marinade. Alternately thread beef and vegetables onto 6 metal skewers, ending with beef. Brush barbecue grid with olive oil. Grill kabobs, on covered grill, over hot coals 6 to 8 minutes for medium-rare or until desired doneness is reached, turning and brushing with reserved marinade halfway through grilling time. *Makes 6 entrée servings*

Nutrients per Serving: Calories: 247 (69% of calories from fat), Total Fat: 19 g, Saturated Fat: 5 g, Cholesterol: 38 mg, Sodium: 233 mg, Carbohydrate: 3 g, Dietary Fiber: 1 g, Protein: 16 g
Dietary Exchanges: 2 Meat, 3 Fat

Pineapple Turkey Kabobs

1½ pounds boneless skinless turkey tenders
2 large red bell peppers
2 cups fresh pineapple chunks
½ cup rice wine or white wine vinegar
¼ cup pickled ginger
2 teaspoons chopped garlic
½ teaspoon black pepper
Olive oil cooking spray

1. Soak 6 wooden skewers in water 20 minutes. Preheat oven to 400°F. Cut turkey into bite-size pieces; place in resealable food storage bag.

2. Cut bell peppers into bite-size chunks. Add bell peppers, pineapple, vinegar, pickled ginger, garlic and black pepper to bag with turkey. Seal bag; turn several times to coat all ingredients. Refrigerate 20 minutes.

3. Spray 11×9-inch baking pan with cooking spray. Assemble 6 skewers by threading pieces of bell pepper, turkey, ginger and pineapple on each. Place in prepared pan; cover with foil. Bake 20 to 25 minutes or until turkey is cooked through. Serve with rice, if desired.   *Makes 6 entrée servings*

Nutrients per Serving: Calories: 171 (5% of calories from fat), Total Fat: 1 g, Saturated Fat: <1 g, Cholesterol: 74 mg, Sodium: 47 mg, Carbohydrate: 11 g, Dietary Fiber: 2 g, Protein: 28 g
Dietary Exchanges: 1 Fruit, 3 Lean Meat

Chicken Breasts Florentine

2 pounds boneless, skinless chicken breasts
¼ cup all-purpose flour
2 eggs, well beaten
⅔ cup seasoned dry bread crumbs
¼ cup BERTOLLI° Olive Oil
1 medium clove garlic, finely chopped
½ cup dry white wine
1 envelope LIPTON° RECIPE SECRETS° Golden Onion
    Soup Mix
1½ cups water
2 tablespoons finely chopped fresh parsley
⅛ teaspoon ground black pepper
    Hot cooked rice pilaf or white rice
    Hot cooked spinach

Dip chicken in flour, then eggs, then bread crumbs.

In 12-inch skillet, heat oil over medium heat and cook chicken until almost done. Remove chicken. Reserve 1 tablespoon drippings. Add garlic and wine to reserved drippings and cook over medium heat 5 minutes. Stir in soup mix thoroughly blended with water; bring to a boil. Return chicken to skillet and simmer covered 10 minutes or until chicken is thoroughly cooked and sauce is slightly thickened. Stir in parsley and pepper. To serve, arrange chicken over hot rice and spinach; garnish as desired. *Makes about 6 entrée servings*

Nutrients per Serving (without rice pilaf or spinach): Calories: 346 (34% of calories from fat), Total Fat: 13 g, Saturated Fat: 2 g, Cholesterol: 158 mg, Sodium: 599 mg, Carbohydrate: 16 g, Dietary Fiber: 1 g, Protein: 39 g
Dietary Exchanges: 1 Starch, 5 Meat

Hearty Lentil Stew

2 tablespoons BERTOLLI® Olive Oil
3 medium carrots, sliced
3 ribs celery, sliced
1 cup lentils
3 cups water, divided
1 envelope LIPTON® RECIPE SECRETS® Savory Herb with
   Garlic Soup Mix*
1 tablespoon cider vinegar or red wine vinegar
   Hot cooked brown rice, couscous or pasta

*Also terrific with LIPTON® RECIPE SECRETS® Onion Mushroom or Onion Soup Mix.

In 3-quart saucepan, heat oil over medium heat and cook carrots and celery, stirring occasionally, 3 minutes. Add lentils and cook 1 minute. Stir in 2 cups water. Bring to a boil over high heat. Reduce heat to low and simmer covered, stirring occasionally, 25 minutes. Stir in soup mix blended with remaining 1 cup water. Simmer covered additional 10 minutes or until lentils are tender. Stir in vinegar. Serve over hot rice.

Makes about 4 entrée servings

Nutrients per Serving (with rice): Calories: 265 (24% of calories from fat), Total Fat: 7 g, Saturated Fat: 1 g, Cholesterol: 0 mg, Sodium: 670 mg, Carbohydrate: 36 g, Dietary Fiber: 16 g, Protein: 15 g
Dietary Exchanges: 2½ Vegetable, 1 Meat, 1 Fat

Roast Pork Chops
with Apple and Cabbage

 3 teaspoons olive oil, divided
½ medium onion, thinly sliced
 1 teaspoon dried thyme
 2 cloves garlic, minced
 4 pork chops (6 to 8 ounces each), 1 inch thick
   Salt and black pepper
¼ cup cider vinegar
 1 tablespoon packed brown sugar
 1 large McIntosh apple, chopped
½ (8-ounce) package shredded coleslaw mix

1. Preheat over to 375°F.

2. Heat 2 teaspoons oil in large ovenproof skillet over medium-high heat until hot. Add onion; cook, covered, 4 to 6 minutes or until tender, stirring often. Add thyme and garlic; cook and stir 30 seconds. Transfer to small bowl; set aside.

3. Add remaining 1 teaspoon oil to same skillet. Sprinkle pork with ⅛ teaspoon salt and pepper. Brown pork 2 minutes on each side. Remove pork from skillet; set aside.

4. Remove skillet from heat. Stir in vinegar, brown sugar and ¼ teaspoon pepper until sugar is dissolved. Add onion mixture, apple and coleslaw mix; do not stir. Top with pork chops. Cover; bake 15 minutes or until pork is barely pink in center.   *Makes 4 entrée servings*

Nutrients per Serving: Calories: 241 (49% of calories from fat),
Total Fat: 13 g, Saturated Fat: 20 g, Cholesterol: 60 mg, Sodium: 66 mg,
Carbohydrate: 13 g, Dietary Fiber: 1 g, Protein: 19 g
Dietary Exchanges: ½ Fruit, 1 Vegetable, 2½ Lean Meat, 1 Fat

Tuscan Vegetable Stew

2 tablespoons olive oil
2 teaspoons minced garlic
1 package (8 ounces) sliced button mushrooms
¼ cup sliced shallots or chopped onion
1 jar (7 ounces) roasted red peppers
1 can (about 14 ounces) Italian-style stewed tomatoes, undrained
1 can (19 ounces) cannellini beans, rinsed and drained
1 bunch fresh basil leaves*
1 tablespoon balsamic or red wine vinegar
  Salt and black pepper
  Grated Romano, Parmesan or Asiago cheese (optional)

*Or, add 2 teaspoons dried basil leaves to stew with tomatoes.

1. Heat oil and garlic in large deep skillet over medium heat. Add mushrooms and shallots; cook and stir 5 minutes.

2. Meanwhile, drain and rinse peppers; cut into 1-inch pieces. Snip tomatoes into small pieces with scissors.

3. Add tomatoes, peppers and beans to skillet; bring to a boil. Reduce heat to medium-low. Cover; simmer 10 minutes.

4. Meanwhile, cut basil leaves into thin strips to measure ¼ cup. Stir basil and vinegar into stew; add salt and black pepper to taste. Serve with cheese, if desired.

Makes 4 entrée servings

Nutrients per Serving: Calories: 235 (33% of calories from fat), Total Fat: 8 g, Saturated Fat: 1 g, Cholesterol: 0 mg, Sodium: 585 mg, Carbohydrate: 30 g, Dietary Fiber: 6 g, Protein: 8 g
Dietary Exchanges: 2 Starch, 2 Fat

Tuscany Cavatelli

16 ounces uncooked cavatelli, penne or ziti pasta
1½ cups seeded diced plum tomatoes
⅔ cup chopped pimiento-stuffed green olives
¼ cup drained capers
2 tablespoons grated Parmesan cheese
2 tablespoons olive oil
2 tablespoons balsamic or red wine vinegar
2 cloves garlic, minced
½ teaspoon black pepper

1. Cook pasta according to package directions, omitting salt. Drain; set aside.

2. Combine tomatoes, olives, capers, cheese, oil, vinegar, garlic and pepper in medium bowl. Stir in pasta until thoroughly coated. Serve warm or at room temperature.

Makes 5 entrée servings

Note: Capers are the small, pea-size buds of flowers from the caper bush. Found mostly in Central America and the Mediterranean, capers add pungency to sauces, dips and relishes. Usually these green buds are pickled and can be found in the condiment section of the supermarket.

Nutrients per Serving: Calories: 452 (21% of calories from fat),
Total Fat: 11 g, Saturated Fat: 2 g, Cholesterol: 2 mg, Sodium: 777 mg,
Carbohydrate: 75 g, Dietary Fiber: 2 g, Protein: 14 g
Dietary Exchanges: 5 Starch, 2 Fat

Tomato Pastina Soup

2 teaspoons olive oil
⅔ cup coarsely chopped green bell pepper
½ cup coarsely chopped onion
½ cup coarsely chopped cucumber
3 cloves garlic, minced
1½ pounds fresh tomatoes, coarsely chopped
1 can (14½ ounces) whole tomatoes, undrained
2 tablespoons red wine vinegar
2 teaspoons ground cumin
1 teaspoon coriander seeds
½ teaspoon black pepper
¼ teaspoon salt
1 ounce uncooked pastina
1 cup water

1. Heat oil in large saucepan over medium heat. Add bell pepper, onion, cucumber and garlic; cook and stir until pepper and onion are tender. Add fresh and canned tomatoes, vinegar, cumin, coriander, black pepper and salt. Bring to a boil. Reduce heat; simmer, covered, 15 minutes. Remove from heat; cool.

2. Place tomato mixture in food processor or blender; process in small batches until smooth. Return to saucepan. Bring to a boil over high heat. Add pasta; cook 4 to 6 minutes or until pasta is tender. Stir in water; transfer to serving bowls.

Makes 6 servings

Nutrients per Serving (¾ cup soup): Calories: 93 (21% of calories from fat), Total Fat: 2 g, Saturated Fat: <1 g, Cholesterol: 0 mg, Sodium: 214 mg, Carbohydrate: 17 g, Dietary Fiber: 3 g, Protein: 3 g
Dietary Exchanges: ½ Starch, 2 Vegetable, ½ Fat

Hearty Bean & Pasta Soup

1 cup uncooked elbow macaroni
2 tablespoons olive oil
1 medium onion, chopped
2 cloves garlic, minced
4 cups water
2 cans (14½ ounces each) reduced-sodium chicken broth
1 jar (26 ounces) marinara sauce
1 can (15 ounces) Great Northern or cannellini beans,
    rinsed and drained
2 teaspoons red wine vinegar
1 pound fresh spinach, chopped
½ cup grated Parmesan cheese (optional)

1. Cook macaroni according to package directions; drain.

2. Meanwhile, heat oil in Dutch oven or large saucepan over medium heat. Add onion and garlic; cook and stir 5 minutes or until onion is tender.

3. Stir in water, broth, marinara sauce and beans; bring to a boil. Reduce heat to low; cook, uncovered, 10 minutes, stirring occasionally. Stir in spinach and cooked pasta; cook 5 minutes. Sprinkle with cheese before serving.

Makes 10 to 12 servings

Nutrients per Serving: Calories: 172 (21% of calories from fat), Total Fat: 4 g, Saturated Fat: 1 g, Cholesterol: 9 mg, Sodium: 560 mg, Carbohydrate: 26 g, Dietary Fiber: 6 g, Protein: 9 g
Dietary Exchanges: 2 Starch, 2 Vegetable, 1 Fat

Roasted Pepper and Avocado Salad

2 red bell peppers
2 orange bell peppers
2 yellow bell peppers
2 ripe avocados, halved, pitted and peeled
3 shallots, thinly sliced
¼ cup FILIPPO BERIO® Extra Virgin Olive Oil
1 clove garlic, crushed
    Finely grated peel and juice of 1 lemon
    Salt and freshly ground black pepper

Place bell peppers on baking sheet. Broil, 4 to 5 inches from heat, 5 minutes on each side or until entire surface of each bell pepper is blistered and blackened slightly. Place bell peppers in paper bag. Close bag; cool 15 to 20 minutes. Cut around cores of bell peppers; twist and remove. Cut bell peppers lengthwise in half. Peel off skin with paring knife; rinse under cold water to remove seeds. Slice bell peppers into ½-inch-thick strips; place in shallow dish. Cut avocados into ¼-inch-thick slices; add to bell peppers. Sprinkle with shallots.

In small bowl, whisk together olive oil, garlic, lemon peel and juice. Pour over bell pepper mixture. Cover; refrigerate at least 1 hour before serving. Season to taste with salt and black pepper.
    Makes 6 servings

Nutrients per Serving (without salt): Calories: 222 (73% of calories from fat), Total Fat: 18 g, Saturated Fat: 2 g, Cholesterol: 0 mg, Sodium: 9 mg, Carbohydrate: 16 g, Dietary Fiber: 6 g, Protein: 3 g
Dietary Exchanges: 3 Vegetable, 3½ Fat

Greek Pasta and Vegetable Salad

⅔ cup uncooked corkscrew macaroni
⅓ cup lime juice
2 tablespoons honey
1 tablespoon olive oil
1 clove garlic, minced
4 cups torn stemmed spinach
1 cup sliced cucumber
½ cup thinly sliced carrot
¼ cup sliced green onions
2 tablespoons crumbled feta cheese
2 tablespoons sliced pitted ripe olives

Prepare macaroni according to package directions, omitting salt; drain. Rinse under cold water; drain. Combine lime juice, honey, oil and garlic in large bowl. Stir in macaroni. Cover; marinate in refrigerator 2 to 24 hours.

Combine spinach, cucumber, carrot, onions, cheese and olives in large bowl. Add macaroni mixture to salad; toss to coat.

Makes 4 main-dish servings

Nutrients per Serving: Calories: 188 (28% of calories from fat), Total Fat: 6 g, Saturated Fat: 1 g, Cholesterol: 3 mg, Sodium: 230 mg, Carbohydrate: 30 g, Dietary Fiber: 2 g, Protein: 5 g
Dietary Exchanges: 1 Starch, 3 Vegetable, 1 Fat

Italian Artichoke and Rotini Salad

4 ounces uncooked whole wheat or tri-colored rotini
   pasta
1 can (14 ounces) quartered artichoke hearts, drained
½ cup (4 ounces) sliced pimientos
1 can (2½ ounces) sliced black olives, drained
2 tablespoons finely chopped yellow onion
2 teaspoons dried basil
1 clove garlic, minced
⅛ teaspoon black pepper
3 tablespoons cider vinegar
1 tablespoon extra-virgin olive oil
¼ teaspoon salt

1. Cook rotini according to package directions, omitting salt
and oil. Meanwhile, combine artichokes, pimientos, olives,
onion, basil, garlic and pepper in medium bowl.

2. Drain pasta in colander; rinse under cold running water to
cool completely. Drain well. Add to artichoke mixture; toss to
blend. Just before serving, combine vinegar, oil and salt; whisk
until well blended. Toss with pasta mixture to coat.

Makes 6 (¾-cup) servings

Nutrients per Serving: Calories: 130 (28% of calories from fat), Total Fat: 4 g,
Saturated Fat: <1 g, Cholesterol: 0 mg, Sodium: 390 mg, Carbohydrate: 21 g,
Dietary Fiber: 5 g, Protein: 5 g
Dietary Exchanges: 1½ Starch, ½ Fat

Lentil and Orzo Pasta Salad

  8 cups water
½ cup uncooked dried lentils, rinsed and sorted
  4 ounces uncooked orzo pasta
1½ cups quartered cherry or grape tomatoes
¾ cup finely chopped celery
½ cup chopped red onion
  2 ounces pitted olives (about 16), coarsely chopped
  3 to 4 tablespoons cider vinegar
  1 tablespoon dried basil
  1 tablespoon olive oil
  1 medium clove garlic, minced
⅛ teaspoon dried red pepper flakes
  4 ounces feta with sun-dried tomatoes and basil

1. Bring water to boil in Dutch oven over high heat. Add lentils; boil 12 minutes.

2. Add orzo; cook 10 minutes or until orzo is just tender. Drain. Rinse under cold water to cool completely. Drain well.

3. Meanwhile, combine remaining ingredients except feta in large bowl; set aside.

4. Add lentil mixture to tomato mixture; toss gently to blend. Add cheese; toss gently. Let stand 15 minutes before serving.

Makes 4 (1⅓-cup) servings

Nutrients per Serving: Calories: 343 (32% of calories from fat),
Total Fat: 13 g, Saturated Fat: 5 g, Cholesterol: 21 mg, Sodium: 470 mg,
Carbohydrate: 44 g, Dietary Fiber: 11 g, Protein: 17 g
Dietary Exchanges: 2½ Starch, 1½ Vegetable, 1 Lean Meat, 1½ Fat

Salmon Salad with Basil Vinaigrette

　　Basil Vinaigrette (recipe follows)
　1 pound asparagus, trimmed
1¼ teaspoons salt, divided
　1 pound salmon fillets
1½ teaspoons olive oil
　¼ teaspoon black pepper
　4 lemon wedges

1. Prepare Basil Vinaigrette. Preheat oven to 400°F or preheat grill to medium-hot. Place 3 inches of water and 1 teaspoon salt in large saucepan or Dutch oven. Bring to boil over high heat. Add asparagus; boil gently 6 to 8 minutes or until asparagus is crisp-tender; drain and set aside.

2. Brush salmon with olive oil. Sprinkle with remaining ¼ teaspoon salt and pepper. Place fish in shallow baking pan; cook 11 to 13 minutes or until fish just begins to flake when tested with fork. (Or, grill on well-oiled grid over medium-hot coals 4 or 5 minutes per side or until fish just begins to flake when tested with fork.)

3. Remove skin from salmon. Break salmon into bite-size pieces. Arrange salmon over asparagus spears on serving plate. Spoon Basil Vinaigrette over salmon. Serve with lemon wedges.

Makes 4 (1½-cup) servings

Basil Vinaigrette

3 tablespoons extra-virgin olive oil
1 tablespoon minced fresh basil
1 tablespoon white wine vinegar
1 small clove garlic, minced
1 teaspoon minced fresh chives
¼ teaspoon black pepper
⅛ teaspoon salt

Combine all ingredients in small bowl; stir until blended.

Makes 4 servings

Nutrients per Serving: Calories: 332 (65% of calories from fat),
Total Fat: 24 g, Saturated Fat: 5 g, Cholesterol: 56 mg, Sodium: 856 mg,
Carbohydrate: 5 g, Dietary Fiber: 2 g, Protein: 25 g
Dietary Exchanges: 1 Vegetable, 3 Lean Meat, 3 Fat

Fresh Pepper Pasta Salad

5 tablespoons olive oil, divided
4 red or yellow bell peppers, seeded and cut into strips
2 cloves garlic, cut into thin slices
3 tablespoons balsamic vinegar
½ teaspoon salt
½ teaspoon black pepper
8 ounces uncooked rotelle pasta
¾ cup fresh basil leaves, cut into thin strips
1½ cups canned chickpeas, rinsed and drained
½ cup grated Parmesan cheese
⅓ cup chopped walnuts
¼ cup sliced green olives (optional)

1. Heat 2 tablespoons oil in large nonstick skillet over medium heat. Add half of bell pepper strips and garlic; cook and stir 2 minutes. Cover; cook 10 minutes or until very soft, stirring occasionally.

2. Place peppers in food processor or blender. Add remaining 3 tablespoons oil, vinegar, salt and black pepper; process until smooth. Cool.

3. Cook pasta according to package directions. Drain. Place in large bowl. Add remaining bell pepper strips and dressing; toss to coat. Cool slightly. Add basil, chickpeas, cheese, walnuts and olives, if desired, to pasta mixture; toss to blend. Serve at room temperature or chilled. *Makes 8 (1-cup) servings*

Nutrients per Serving: Calories: 313 (40% of calories from fat),
Total Fat: 14 g, Saturated Fat: 2 g, Cholesterol: 4 mg, Sodium: 360 mg,
Carbohydrate: 38 g, Dietary Fiber: 4 g, Protein: 9 g
Dietary Exchanges: 2½ Starch, ½ Lean Meat, 2 Fat

Mediterranean-Style Roasted Vegetables

1½ pounds red potatoes
  1 tablespoon plus 1½ teaspoons olive oil, divided
  1 red bell pepper
  1 yellow or orange bell pepper
  1 small red onion
  2 cloves garlic, minced
  ½ teaspoon salt
  ¼ teaspoon black pepper
  1 tablespoon balsamic or red wine vinegar
  ¼ cup chopped fresh basil leaves

1. Preheat oven to 425°F. Spray large shallow metal roasting pan with nonstick olive oil cooking spray. Cut potatoes into 1½-inch chunks; place in pan. Drizzle 1 tablespoon oil over potatoes; toss to coat. Bake 10 minutes.

2. Cut bell peppers into 1½-inch pieces. Cut onion into ½-inch wedges. Add bell peppers and onion to pan. Drizzle remaining 1½ teaspoons oil over vegetables; sprinkle with garlic, salt and black pepper. Toss well to coat. Return to oven; bake 18 to 20 minutes or until vegetables are browned and tender, stirring once.

3. Transfer to large serving bowl. Drizzle vinegar over vegetables; toss to coat. Add basil; toss again. Serve warm or at room temperature with additional black pepper, if desired.

Makes 6 side-dish servings

Nutrients per Serving: Calories: 170 (19% of calories from fat), Total Fat: 4 g, Saturated Fat: <1 g, Cholesterol: 0 mg, Sodium: 185 mg, Carbohydrate: 33 g, Dietary Fiber: 1 g, Protein: 3 g
Dietary Exchanges: 2 Starch, ½ Fat

Barley and Wild Rice Pilaf

2 tablespoons olive oil, divided
1 medium onion, chopped
1 cup uncooked pearl barley
½ cup uncooked wild rice, rinsed and drained
3 cloves garlic, minced
4 cups fat-free, reduced-sodium chicken broth
1 large red bell pepper, cut into ¼-inch pieces
3 ounces fresh mushrooms, thinly sliced
½ cup frozen green peas, thawed
½ cup shredded carrot
1 teaspoon dried oregano

1. Heat 1 tablespoon oil in large saucepan over medium heat. Cook and stir onion about 10 minutes or until tender. Add barley, rice and garlic; cook and stir over medium heat 1 minute.

2. Stir in chicken broth. Bring to a boil. Reduce heat; simmer, covered, about 1 hour or until barley and rice are tender.

3. Heat remaining 1 tablespoon oil in large skillet over medium-high heat. Cook and stir bell pepper, mushrooms, peas, carrot and oregano 5 to 6 minutes or until vegetables are tender. Stir bell pepper mixture into rice mixture.

Makes 8 side-dish servings

Nutrients per Serving: Calories: 180 (19% of calories from fat), Total Fat: 4 g, Saturated Fat: 1 g, Cholesterol: 0 mg, Sodium: 35 mg, Carbohydrate: 32 g, Dietary Fiber: 6 g, Protein: 6 g
Dietary Exchanges: 2 Starch, 1 Vegetable, 1 Fat

Country Green Beans with Turkey Ham

  2 teaspoons olive oil
  ¼ cup minced onion
  1 clove garlic, minced
  1 pound fresh green beans, rinsed and drained
  1 cup chopped fresh tomatoes
  6 slices (2 ounces) thinly sliced low-fat smoked turkey
      ham
  1 tablespoon chopped fresh marjoram
  2 teaspoons chopped fresh basil
  ⅛ teaspoon black pepper
  ¼ cup herbed croutons

1. Heat oil in medium saucepan over medium heat. Add onion and garlic; cook and stir about 4 minutes or until onion is tender. Reduce heat to low.

2. Add green beans, tomatoes, turkey ham, marjoram, basil and pepper. Cook about 10 minutes, stirring occasionally, until liquid from tomatoes is absorbed and beans are tender.

3. Transfer mixture to serving dish. Top with croutons.

Makes 4 side-dish servings

Nutrients per Serving: Calories: 100 (27% of calories from fat), Total Fat: 3 g, Saturated Fat: 1 g, Cholesterol: 12 mg, Sodium: 194 mg, Carbohydrate: 14 g, Dietary Fiber: 4 g, Protein: 6 g
Dietary Exchanges: 3 Vegetable, ½ Fat

Orzo with Spinach and Red Pepper

4 ounces uncooked orzo
   Nonstick olive oil cooking spray
1 teaspoon olive oil
1 medium red bell pepper, diced
3 cloves garlic, minced
1 package (10 ounces) frozen chopped spinach, thawed
   and squeezed dry
¼ cup grated Parmesan cheese
½ teaspoon finely chopped fresh oregano or basil leaves
   (optional)
¼ teaspoon lemon pepper

1. Prepare orzo according to package directions; drain and set aside.

2. Spray large nonstick skillet with cooking spray. Heat skillet over medium-high heat until hot; add oil, tilting skillet to coat bottom. Add bell pepper and garlic; cook and stir 2 to 3 minutes or until bell pepper is crisp-tender. Add orzo and spinach; stir until well mixed and heated through. Remove from heat; stir in Parmesan cheese, oregano, if desired, and lemon pepper. Garnish as desired.

Makes 6 side-dish servings

Nutrients per Serving: Calories: 116 (19% of calories from fat), Total Fat: 3 g, Saturated Fat: 1 g, Cholesterol: 3 mg, Sodium: 152 mg, Carbohydrate: 19 g, Dietary Fiber: 2 g, Protein: 6 g
Dietary Exchanges: 1 Starch, 1 Vegetable, ½ Fat

RECIPE INDEX

The publisher would like
to thank the companies
and organizations
listed below for the use
of their recipes in this
publication.

Cabot® Creamery
Cooperative
Filippo Berio® Olive Oil
Unilever

GENERAL INDEX

A

Acetic acid, 65, 77, 88–89, 97
Age spots, 67
Aging, 69, 82–84
Ajoene, 12
Allicin
  benefits of, 32, 37, 39
  cooking garlic and, 27, 61
  described, 12
Antioxidants, 13, 22–25, 69
Appetite problems, 67
Apple cider vinegar, 90, 96–99
Arteriosclerosis, 13
Arthritis, 30
Artichoke garlic, 50
Asthma, 10, 30, 67
Atherosclerosis, 13, 118
Athlete's foot, 34, 67, 76
Autoimmune disorders, 124–125

B

Bacteria, 27–29, 84–85
Balsamic vinegar, 83, 91–94
Beer vinegar, 96
Berry stains, 105
Bladder problems, 10, 67
Blood clotting, 67
Blood pressure
  garlic and, 10, 25–26
  olive oil and, 122–123
  vinegar and, 67, 80–81
Bronchitis, 10
Butter, 113
Buttermilk, 104

C

Calcium, 24, 68, 73–74, 77–78
Cancer
  garlic and, 35–39
  olive oil and, 125, 127–128
  vinegar and, 69
Candy, making, 104
Cane vinegar, 95
Canning, 104
Canola oil, 113
Cholesterol
  dietary fats and, 110–111, 130
  garlic and, 18–22
  in heart disease, 15–18
  numbers associated with, 17
  olive oil and, 115–120, 135
  vinegar and, 67, 68, 80–81
Circulation, 67
Coconut oil, 113
Coconut vinegar, 96
Cold-pressed olive oil, 140
Colds
  garlic and, 10, 30, 31, 32
  vinegar and, 67, 75
Colic, 10
Companion planting, 55
Complementary medicine research, 70
Constipation, 10, 67
Corn oil, 113
Corns, 35
Coughs, 10, 67, 75

D

Dandruff, 10, 67
Deodorizers, 105
Depression, 67
Diabetes
  garlic and, 10, 15
  inflammation and, 126
  olive oil and, 129–130
  vinegar and, 68, 78–80
Diarrhea, 67
Dietary fats, 109–115, 146. *See also specific types.*
Digestive problems, 67, 75
Dizziness, 67
Dysentery, 10

E

E. coli, in vinegar, 90, 100
Ear infections, 10, 42, 67
Eczema, 10, 67
Eggs, cooking, 103
Elephant garlic, 53
Essential fatty acids, 114–115, 146
Estate olive oils, 145
Expeller-pressed olive oil, 140–141
Eyes, sore or tired, 67

F

Fatigue, 67
Fevers, 10
Fibrinolysis, 13
Fish, cooking, 103
Flatulence, 10
Flu, 10

Food poisoning, 67
Free radicals, 69, 117, 122

G

Gallbladder problems, 10, 67
Garlic
  ailments treated with, 10
  amount recommended, 39, 45–47
  blood pressure and, 25–26
  cancer and, 35–39
  cholesterol and, 18–22
  cooking with, 59–61
  diabetes and, 15
  forms of, 20–21
  growing, 53–57
  heart disease and, 12–26
  history and lore of, 7–12, 28
  infections and, 26–35, 42
  inflammation and, 30
  nutrients in, 40
  pickled, 102
  safety of, 41–43
  storing, 57–59
  varieties of, 49–53
  weight control and, 39
Garlic festivals, 51
Garlic supplements, 43–47
Giardia lamblia, 31–33
Gilroy Garlic Festival, 51
Gum disease, 34

H

H. pylori, 37
Hair problems, 10, 67
Hands, washing, 105
Hardneck garlic, 50–53
Hay fever, 67
HDL cholesterol. See Cholesterol.
Headaches, 67
Hearing problems, 67
Heartburn, 67
Heart disease
  cholesterol in, 15–18
  described, 12–15
  garlic and, 22–26
  olive oil and, 115–123
  terms defined, 13–14
  vinegar and, 68, 80–81
Herbal vinegars, 99–102
Hiccups, 67
Homocysteine, 13
Hyperlipidemia, 13

I

Indigestion, 10
Infections, 10, 26–35. See also Ear infections.
Infertility, 10
Inflammation, 30, 123–127
Insect bites or stings, 10, 35, 67, 76
Insomnia, 10, 67
Insulin resistance, 78–80
Intestinal worms, 10

J

Joint pain, 67

K

Kidney problems, 67

L

Labels
  nutrition information, 112, 117, 131
  olive oil extraction information, 140–141
  organic certification, 149
Lactose intolerance, 77
LDL cholesterol. See Cholesterol.
Leg cramps, 67
Linoleic acid, 146
Lipids, 13
Lite olive oil, 149–150
Liver problems, 10
Liver spots, 67

M

Macronutrients
  in garlic, 40
  in vinegar, 72
Malt vinegar, 95
Meat tenderizer, 103
Mediterranean diet, 120, 133–135
Memory problems, 10
Menstrual problems, 10
Metabolic syndrome, 121
Metabolism problems, 67
Minerals. See also Calcium.
  in garlic, 40
  in vinegar, 72–73
Monounsaturated fat
  benefits of, 121–122, 129–130
  described, 110
  in olive oil, 112, 146

Mother of vinegar, 98
Muscle strains, 67

N

Nasal congestion, 67, 75
Nitric oxide, 14, 118, 119
NSAIDs, 125, 126
Nutrition labels, 112, 117, 131

O

Obesity. See Weight control.
Oleic acid, 127–128, 143, 146
Oleocanthal, 126–127
Olive oil
    acidity of, 143
    ailments treated with, 108–109
    blood pressure and, 122–123
    buying, 147, 153
    cancer and, 125, 127–128
    cholesterol and, 115–120, 135
    color of, 138, 150–151
    contraindications for, 108
    cooking with, 156–160
    diabetes and, 129–130
    dietary fat in, 112–115, 146
    freezing, 154
    geographic origins of, 144–145
    grades of, 145–150
    heart disease and, 115–123

Olive oil (continued)
    history and lore of, 106–107, 109, 139
    inflammation and, 123–127
    labels on, 140–141
    nutrition content of, 134, 146
    production of, 137–144
    quality standards for, 142–144
    shelf life of, 155–156
    storing, 151–156
    taste of, 142
    weight control and, 130–135
Olives
    oil content of, 128, 135
    polyphenol content of, 137
Olive trees, 107, 109
Omega fatty acids, 114–115, 146
Organic olive oil, 149
Osteoarthritis, 30
Osteoporosis, 67, 69
Oxidation, 14, 122

P

Palm kernel oil, 113
Palm oil, 113
Paralysis, 10
Pastry, making, 105
Peanut oil, 113
Pectin, 68, 74
Periodontitis, 34
Pesticides, on produce, 84–85
Phenolic compounds, 115–120, 124, 130
Pickling, 102, 104
Plaque, 14–15, 22–25, 117, 125

Polyphenolic compounds, 116–120, 130, 137, 138
Polyunsaturated fat, 110, 114–115, 124, 146
Pomace, 141, 148–149
Porcelain garlic, 52
Potassium, 68, 74
Potatoes, cooking, 104
Prescription medications, garlic and, 41
Produce
    including in diet, 82–84
    washing, 84–85
Prostaglandins, 114
Purple stripe garlic, 52–53

R

Rabies, 10
Raisin vinegar, 96
Rancid oils, 152
Refined olive oils, 148
Rheumatism, 10
Rice vinegar, 94
Rocambole, 51–52

S

Safflower oil, 113
Saturated fat, 80–81, 110
Scabies, 10
Seizures, 10
Shortening, 113
Silverskin garlic, 50
Sinus problems, 10
Sodium, 80–81
Softneck garlic, 49–50
Solvent-extracted olive oil, 141
Sore throat, 67
Soybean oil, 113

Stomach upset, 67, 75
Storage methods
  garlic, 57–59
  olive oil, 151–156
  vinegar, 103
Stroke, 80–81
Sulfur compounds, 7
Sunburn, 67
Sunflower oil, 113
Supplements
  garlic, 43–47
  vinegar, 86–87

T

Tallow, 113
Trans fats, 80–81,
  111–112, 124
Tremors, 10
Triglycerides, 18, 21,
  115
Tuberculosis, 10
Typhoid, 10

U

Ulcers, 10
Urinary tract infec-
  tions, 67
USDA Web site, 104

V

Vacuum-extracted olive
  oil, 140

Vegetable oils, fat in,
  113
Vegetables
  including in diet,
    82–84
  washing, 84–85
Vinegar
  acidity of, 97
  aging and, 82–84
  ailments treated
    with, 66–69,
    75–76
  blood pressure and,
    80–81
  calcium absorption
    and, 77–78
  cholesterol and,
    80–81
  cooking with, 81–84,
    92, 95, 103–104
  diabetes and, 78–80
  flavor-infused,
    99–102
  heart disease and,
    80–81
  history and lore of,
    28, 63–66
  homemade, 96–99,
    100
  household uses for,
    105
  mother of vinegar,
    98

Vinegar *(continued)*
  nutrients in, 71–74
  production of,
    64–65, 88–89
  storing, 103
  stroke and, 80–81
  varieties of, 89–96
Vinegar supplements,
  86–87
Virgin olive oils,
  145–147, 158
Vitamins, in garlic, 40

W

Walnut oil, 113
Warts, 34–35
Weight control
  garlic and, 39
  olive oil and,
    130–135
  vinegar and, 68
White vinegar, 89
Whooping cough, 10
Wines, 63–64
Wine vinegar, 91
Wounds, 34, 35

Y

Yeast infections, 33, 67